THE MATURE MAN'S GUIDE TO STYLE

Also by Bill Gale

THE WONDERFUL WORLD OF WALKING

THE MATURE MAN'S GUIDE TO STYLE

Diet, Exercise, Fashion, and Grooming for a Man's Best Years

BILL GALE

WILLIAM MORROW AND COMPANY, INC.
New York   *1980*

Copyright © 1980 by William Gale

All rights reserved. No part of this book may be reproduced or utilized in any form or by any means, electronic or mechanical, including photocopying, recording or by any information storage and retrieval system, without permission in writing from the Publisher. Inquiries should be addressed to William Morrow and Company, Inc., 105 Madison Ave., New York, N. Y. 10016.

Library of Congress Cataloging in Publication Data

Gale, Bill.
   The mature man's guide to style.

   Includes index.
   1. Grooming for men.   2. Middle aged men—Health and hygiene.   3. Men's clothing.   I. Title.
RA777.8.G32   646.7′2   80-13843
ISBN 0-688-03688-0

Printed in the United States of America

First Edition

1 2 3 4 5 6 7 8 9 10

BOOK DESIGN BY MICHAEL MAUCERI

This book is dedicated to men everywhere who refuse to be intimidated by the calendar, and begin each day with enthusiasm and verve.

Contents

Introduction   9

Part One

  LOOKING LIKE A MILLION   11
    For Healthy, More Manageable Hair   13
    For Clear, Firm Skin   31
    For Strong, Nimble Legs and Feet   55
    For a Straight, Pain-Free Back and Firm,
      Flat Stomach   61
    For Clear, Youthful-Looking Eyes   67
    For Smooth Hands and Strong Nails   73
    For a Winning Smile   77

Part Two

  LOOKING . . . AND *FEELING* LIKE A MILLION   83
    How to Conquer Stress   85
    Eating Well   91
    Exercising Regularly   109

Part Three

  DRESSING RICH   143

A Gallery of Men Who Look and Feel Like a Million

    Hardy Amies   193
    Warren Anderson   196
    Bill Blass   198
    Jeffrey Butler   201
    C. Carson Conrad   204
    Douglas Fairbanks, Jr.   208
    William Fine   211
    Gerard William Ford   214
    Frank Gifford   216
    Mark Hatfield   219
    Gaylord Hauser   222

Jim Jensen	225
Jim Kimberly	228
Bill Loock	231
David Mahoney	234
Charles Percy	237
Louis Polk	240
Bobby Short	243
Lowell Thomas	246
John Weitz	249
Index	253

Introduction

When a man reaches 40 or 50 he simply doesn't want to be old. . . . He wants all his clothes shapely, tailored, fitted to the figure. This man is also open to something for his face. He's open to something for his hair. He's open to something for his body. That's what's happening.

—CHARLES REVSON, chairman of Revlon,
Life, August 13, 1965

Right on, as they used to say back then.

Still, genes do count for something. They determine how tall you are, how thick your hair is, and, more important, how long you'll keep it. But as you age and your body mechanics change, maintenance counts for a lot, too.

The man who knows how to take prime care of himself can often look more attractive at forty or fifty than he did at twenty-five, for the simple reason that he knows himself so much better and, as a result, is more comfortable with himself. In short, he knows what makes him tick.

And that's what this book is all about: how to correct what's wrong; how to enhance what's right; how to look your *best*. No man should settle for less.

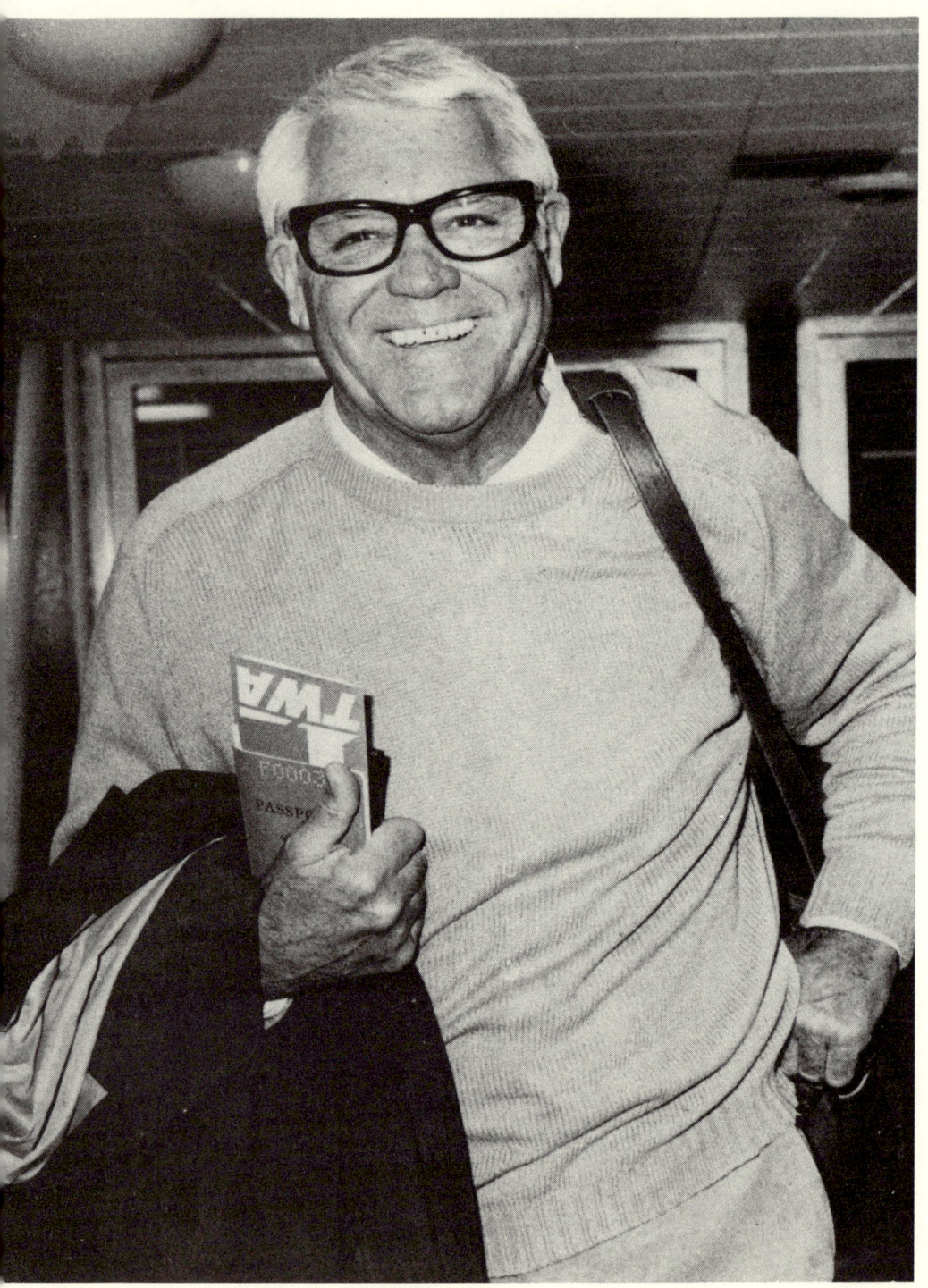

Cary Grant at seventy-plus—and looking like a million.
PHOTO COURTESY OF WIDE WORLD PHOTOS.

Part One

LOOKING LIKE A MILLION

For Healthy, More Manageable Hair

FACT AND FICTION

Hair is a major concern for a man. Attractive, healthy-looking hair has sex appeal and gives a man an air of presence. But when he starts to lose his hair, he feels he's saying good-bye to his youth—even if he's twenty-five at the time.

It's significant, I think, that when America's rebellious young sparked the nationwide rumble of the sixties sometimes referred to as the Youthquake, they let their hair grow long. What better way to demonstrate upmanship? There are, after all, some 15 to 17 million bald men in the United States. Not all of them are totally bald, of course, but all are showing signs of hair loss: hairline recession; bald spot on the crown; thinning over the top of the scalp. It's called male-pattern baldness. And if a man is going to become bald, he's usually well on his way by age thirty. "Don't trust anybody over thirty," the kids chanted from under bushels of hair.

Ironically, despite man's traditional preoccupation with hair, there's still an incredible amount of misinformation circulating about it. You no doubt remember when it was thought that wetting your comb would dry out your hair and that frequent shampooing was considered a sure way to lose it. Now we know better. Water doesn't damage hair, and you have nothing to fear from daily shampooing—even with a medicated shampoo. But some myths die hard.

Hair is an appendage of your skin. Every part of your body, except the palms of your hands, the soles of your feet, and your lips, is covered with hair follicles, which are nourished by the bloodstream. Ergo, improved circulation means improved hair, and revving up circulation via scalp massage with fingers or vibrator is one way to prevent baldness. Right? *Wrong.*

The late Bernarr Macfadden, publisher and very likely the most ornate personality since Teddy Roosevelt, was a strong advocate of daily scalp massage. "To massage the scalp once a week, as is sometimes done, is not enough," he wrote back in 1949, recommending that a man massage his scalp five or ten minutes every day. "Pinch-

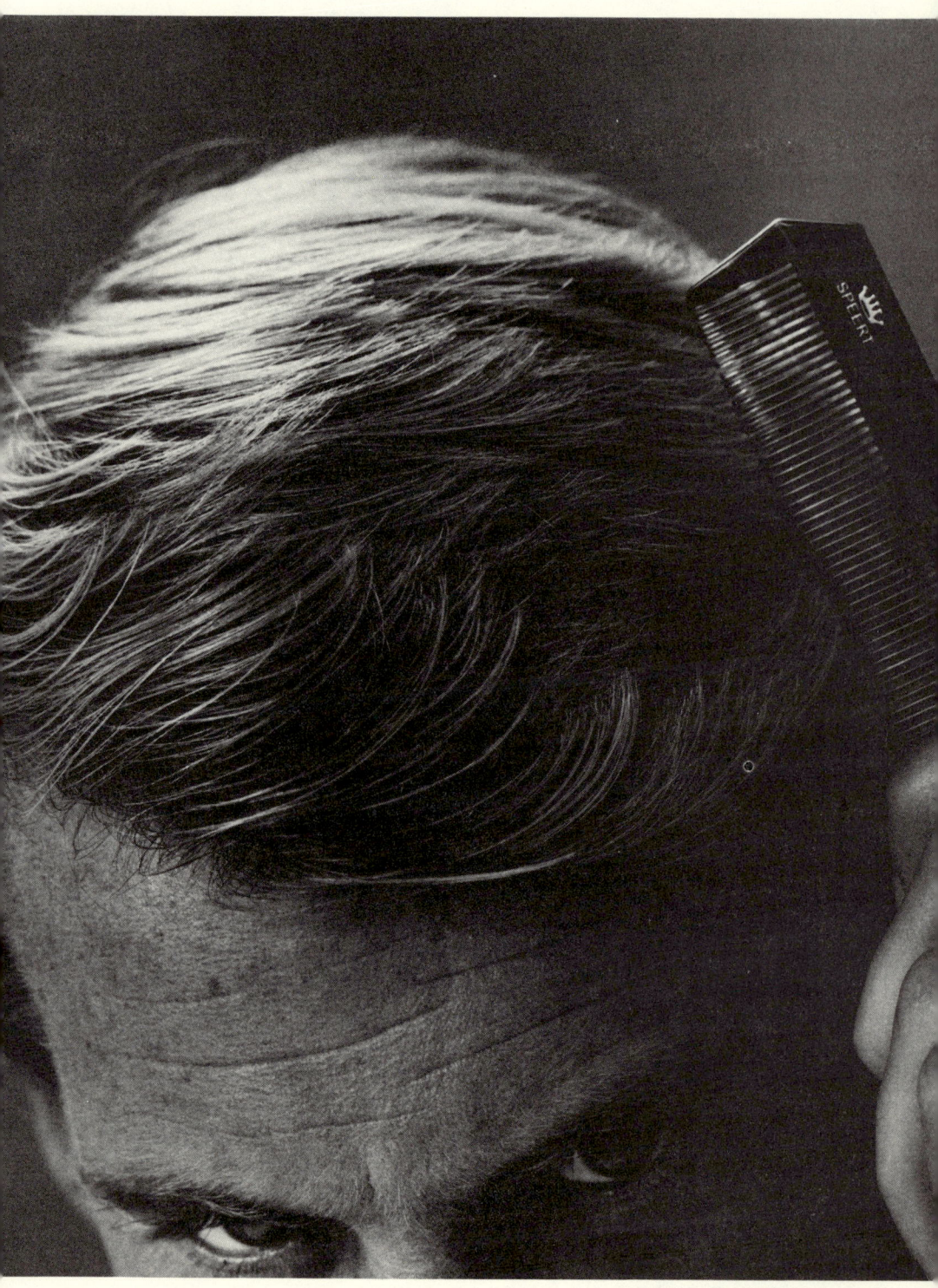

PHOTO BY ROBERT EPSTEIN.

ing and kneading movements should be included." Past eighty and with a leonine head of hair, Macfadden was parachuting out of airplanes and flexing his still-taut muscles in bare-torso publicity pictures. The new husband of a forty-four-year-old widow, he was also asserting his belief that virility should improve with age. So under the circumstances, it wasn't exactly easy to discount his claim that scalp massage was good for hair. A lot of men took it up, and a lot of men are still massaging their scalps in the mistaken belief that a tight scalp is a contributing factor to hair loss because it blunts circulation. I've even heard of a famous film actor who prefaces his daily scalp massage by dunking his head into a bucket of cold water—a fast way, he evidently figures, to stimulate circulation and make his scalp even more pliable.

"Baldness is not due to poor circulation," states Dr. Ronald E. Sherman, a New York dermatologist. "Massage and the pulling of the hair can injure hair follicles." Furthermore, Dr. Richard Gibbs, another prominent New York dermatologist, says that the blood supply is adequate in most balding cases. In fact, it's generally believed that the scalp, bald or hairy, receives more blood than it needs. The myth that a tight scalp contributes to thinning hair and baldness is perpetuated largely by so-called hair specialists offering salon treatments that start with a circulation-stimulating massage of the neck, shoulders, and head that feels good but does absolutely nothing for the health of the hair.

Dermatologists further maintain that vigorous brushing can injure hair follicles. Brush to groom your hair, *not* to exercise it, is their advice. According to Dr. Sherman, brushing hair is rather like brushing fabric: Too much, and it wears out, the brushing action shearing the hair shafts.

CARE AND FEEDING OF YOUR HAIR

You can't nourish your hair follicles by rubbing something into your scalp. And with that truism established, let's move on to the subject of what, if anything, certain foods and vitamin supplements can do to stimulate hair growth.

Are there such things as vitamins for the hair? All the dermatologists and nutritionists I spoke to say no. Yet enough men apparently hope there are to enable one purveyor of vitamins for the hair to run full-page advertisements in national magazines that warn, "You could be stuffing your body and starving your hair." Covering that ground in his book *All About Hair* (Wallingford Press), Dr. Herbert S. Feinberg says, "Whatever hair restorative claim is made for a vitamin or mineral, chances are it's either meaningless for humans in general or anyone's specific hair problem in particular."

Well then, are there foods that nourish the hair follicles? Dr. Robert Giller, a nutritionist with a medical degree from the University of Illinois Medical School and a member of the International Academy of Preventive Medicine, says that he doesn't know of any foods that have an effect on hair growth. And if there were, "they wouldn't be the same for everybody." His advice is to eat wisely—a balanced diet—and that's that so far as diet and the health of your hair are concerned. Only a diet seriously lacking in some essential nutrient can really harm hair—a crash diet, for example, that eliminates protein. Beyond such extreme examples, nutritional deficiency is rarely a cause of hair loss in this country.

Hair is mostly protein (about 97 percent), but it doesn't follow that protein-enriched shampoos and hair-grooming products contribute to the health of hair. Such products don't really contain protein. They're made with compounds derived from protein found in animal tissue, not from keratin, the protein found in human hair. What these protein derivatives can do for hair, however, is to fill in the opening in the hair shaft, so that the hair looks and feels somewhat thicker. But in no way can a so-called protein-enriched shampoo have a lasting effect on the condition of your hair.

Without exception, Dr. Giller urges his patients to eliminate or at least cut down on smoking and alcohol consumption. Cigarette smokers, he says, have higher rates of disability of all kinds and more chronic diseases than nonsmokers, and alcohol interferes with and inhibits the action of many vitamins—not to mention its effect on the liver. But does that mean that tobacco and alcohol have any effect on hair? *No.*

All this brings us back to the tight scalp theory, which maintains that unless the skin of your scalp is as flexible as the skin on your forehead, you're in trouble. The champions of this theory also contend that smoking and drinking impede circulation and therefore deprive follicles of proper nourishment—result: *starved* hair. But as already noted, today's dermatologists disagree. Dr. Gibbs flatly states, "The consumption of alcohol has no effect on scalp and hair at all."

In some quarters, however, there has been considerable interest in the fact that so many of the alcoholics who populate the skid rows of this nation appear to have exceptionally thick hair. I know for years I've been fascinated by the splendid hairlines of many of the men seen on the Bowery, New York City's legendary skid row. So I was intrigued to learn that a few years ago a psychologist by the name of George De Leon conducted what he called "a scientific examination of booze, bums, and hair." He recalled that almost without exception, the alcoholics he had observed over the years had "hair that wouldn't quit." He decided, with the aid of some undergraduates in the university where he taught, actually to "test the hypothesis that booze grows hair."

They observed and interviewed Bowery derelicts and an equal number of men De Leon called sterlings—professional men who were either nondrinkers or purely social drinkers. While he found that older men in both groups contained a greater proportion of hair losers, De Leon discovered the differences between the groups "fascinating," with the derelicts aged forty-one to fifty-five actually showing a slight decrease of hair loss, and only 44 percent of the derelicts past age fifty-five showing signs of balding, compared to about 80 percent of the sterlings in the same age-group. All this led him to conclude that there is no doubt that the skid row alcoholic simply keeps his hair. Reporting on his findings in the October 1977 issue of *Psychology Today*, the psychologist wrote: "It must be the alcohol and some resulting biochemical activity. It happens, since completing the study, that I've learned that medical literature does point to some interaction between liver damage, alcohol metabolism, the female hormone estrogen, hair growth and retention. Seems reasonable to me."

Dr. Richard Rivlin, professor of medicine and chief of nutrition at the Cornell University Medical College, says that there is a lot of experimental evidence in support of the fact that chronic alcohol patients with liver cirrhosis have hormonal disturbances. Since the presence of the male hormone accounts for most cases of baldness, it is believed that the lowered level of male hormones may result in less baldness and sometimes in actual atrophy of the testes. "Libido is often reduced in alcoholic patients with liver disease," notes Dr. Rivlin. So, if the one way a man can keep his hair is to risk cirrhosis of the liver (not to mention loss of libido), better baldness, especially today, when we can quite literally grow new hair without having to take to drink—or celibacy—as you'll see a few pages farther on.

Shampoo

Discussing the subject of alcohol and hair retention, Dr. Gibbs has only this to say: "It proves that dirt is not a factor in loss of hair." In other words, how often you wash your hair is really an aesthetic consideration; unclean hair is not necessarily unhealthy hair. On the other hand, you don't risk baldness if you prefer to shampoo your hair every day. How often you shampoo is up to you, but it stands to reason that an oily scalp needs more frequent shampooing than a dry scalp. And while some men have a so-called normal scalp, neither dry nor oily, most don't.

Hair itself does not have oil glands, and a dry or oily condition depends on whether the sebaceous glands of the scalp are producing too little or too much sebum. No matter. There are shampoos specially formulated for dry and oily hair, and between shampoos there are simple ways to control the condition.

A dry scalp, for instance (sometimes called chapped hair), can be lubricated with a cream- or oil-based pomade or hair groom. Brylcreem is one such product. But a dry look, not bone-dry but one that doesn't look greasy, is desirable today. One way to keep a dry scalp nicely lubricated without your resorting to products that the competition sneeringly refers to as greasy kid stuff is the old-time hot-oil treatment. Apply it before you shampoo, and your hair will look and feel more nearly normal—that is, soft and only slightly oily.

> Heat up some mineral oil, castor oil, or plain cooking oil in a small saucepan. Then, using a comb, section your hair, and with a cotton ball or sterile gauze pad, rub the warm oil into your scalp. Wrap your head in a warm towel, leave it on for fifteen to twenty minutes, and then shampoo. Rinse well, taking care to remove all surface oil.

An oily scalp can often do with daily washing. Still, without shampooing every day, you can blot up some excess oil by simply dampening a cotton ball or sterile gauze pad with rubbing alcohol or witch hazel and dabbing your scalp with it. A shorter haircut helps too, for it reduces the hair's ability to collect oil. And sometimes simply rinsing your hair with cool water will remove enough surface oil so that you can delay shampooing a day or two.

Many men today are using hand-held dryers so they can style their hair while they dry it. To avoid singeing the hair, keep the nozzle of the dryer at least six inches from your scalp, and keep it moving around your head. You've undoubtedly read that an estimated one out of five commercial hair dryers has an asbestos insulator that discharges asbestos particles purported to be cancer-causing, so when buying your dryer, look for one that states clearly that it does *not* have such an insulator.

If you have an oily scalp and use a dryer, put it on a lower setting since too much heat leads to perspiration, which, in turn, will stimulate your already overactive sebaceous glands. If you have a dry scalp condition, I don't recommend you use a dryer any more than I think you should expose your head to the drying effects of summer sun. Settle instead for a soft, thirsty towel. Don't rub your scalp with it, but gently use it to squeeze the rinse water from your hair. Hair is weaker and easily damaged when wet, a fact which makes me wary of shampooing in the shower, for it seems to me that water pounding out of the shower nozzle onto the scalp is hardly the kindly treatment that dermatologists recommend for hair. Furthermore, a shower is a brisk, hearty experience that rather encourages a man to scrub away at his scalp, and that can mean ripping and tearing the hair. While I couldn't find one doctor who would come right out and advise against shampooing in the shower, Dr. Gibbs did allow that it presented "no problem for normal hair." Since thinning hair is not, at least in my opinion, "normal" hair, I recommend that you play it safe and do your shampooing outside the shower.

No matter where you choose to shampoo, gently work the shampoo into your hair, using the cushions of your fingertips, taking care not to scratch your scalp with your nails.

Comb and Brush

The best time to comb your hair is immediately after shampooing, when it's still rather damp; hair is most manageable then.

Your comb and brush should always be as impeccably clean as your just washed hair, so clean them before each shampooing. To clean your comb, soak it for about fifteen minutes in warm, soapy water or a solution of warm water mixed with a few tablespoons of ammonia (if your comb is aluminum, avoid ammonia; it stains the metal). Scrub the comb with a nailbrush until it's thoroughly clean, and then rinse it in cold water. Stand it in a glass or jar to dry.

To clean your brush, place it, bristles down, in warm, soapy water (hot water softens bristles) or warm water mixed with a little ammonia. After about fifteen minutes, rinse it in clear, cold water, shake away the excess water, and then let it dry out on a towel, bristles down, in a warm, dry place.

While on the subject of combs and brushes, I suggest a comb that's sturdy, yet flexible, one with rounded teeth that won't scratch your scalp. When combing, remember to keep your comb in your hair and away from your scalp—it's your hair you're combing. When it comes to selecting a brush, choose one made with natural bristles. Stiff nylon bristles are harsh and tend to wear the hair out. The best brushes I know are actually a combination of mostly natural bristles combined with some synthetic ones and rooted in a rubber cushion. Made in Great Britain, they carry the Mason Pearson brand name.

Conditioners

Some shampoos—even certain medicated ones—have built-in conditioners, but many don't. If you're hell-bent on using a conditioner, you may have to buy one as a separate product or create one of your own.

What does a conditioner do? It coats the hair shaft with a film to give it more body, which makes the hair more manageable while adding some measure of shine.

Besides the commercial conditioner, there are some proved homegrown varieties, for example, the hot-oil treatment for dry hair already described. And for oily hair, there's beer—stale beer. In lieu of a can or bottle of beer that's been opened for, say, a day, you can open a fresh can or bottle, heat it in a pan, and then let it cool. When you're finished shampooing, rinse out the shampoo residue, pour on the beer, and gently work it into your hair. After about ten minutes, rinse.

Henna is another first-rate conditioner. Now I think I probably know your reaction to the idea of using henna. You're recalling the ladies who, back in the twenties and thirties, used it to dye their hair a shade of red so unmistakably the handiwork of henna that there was no other way to describe the shade than to tag it henna red, which was somewhere between the shade of iodine in the shade and burnt orange in the sun. That's not the kind of henna we're talking about here. This is a neutral, or natural, henna that comes from the relatively colorless stem of the Middle Eastern plant called the lawsonia, rather than from its leaves, the source of red henna. As a result, it doesn't change the color of hair. Its action is physical, rather than chemical, for it coats the hair shaft with vegetable matter which adds body while imparting shine. Unlike the hot-oil treatment or the stale-beer rinse, however, this is a conditioning treatment that demands professional application at least until you've gotten the hang of it and can follow product directions to the letter. A professional henna treatment costs somewhere in the neighborhood of $25 to $30, but the added body and shine are said to last for about three months.

DANDRUFF

No one knows yet the cause of dandruff, but what is known is that it has a tendency to be inherited, that it isn't contagious, that more men suffer from it than women do, and that while there is no known cure, the condition can be controlled.

Dermatologists call the condition seborrhea. When this flaking of the scalp (often but not always accompanied by itching) is so severe that not only the scalp but the skin around nose and ears also becomes red and blotchy, dermatologists call that seborrheic dermatitis. While a medicated shampoo is usually enough to control ordinary dandruff, when the condition becomes aggravated, it's time to consult a doctor.

A dry scalp produces dry, saltlike flakes, while an oily scalp produces waxy flakes. Not surprisingly, the dry, saltlike flakes are usually the itchy ones. No matter, for there are medicated antidandruff shampoos specially made for dry and oily scalps, and you needn't be concerned about using yours every day if you find it necessary. Thin, oily hair—with or without the bother of dandruff—needs frequent shampooing since it tends to separate, mat down, and look stringy. And no matter what your shampoo cycle is, always rinse thoroughly, for leftover shampoo not only dulls hair but soon causes flaking as well. A flake's a flake whether it's the result of dandruff or coagulated shampoo, so rinse until the water is crystal-clear, and then rinse one more time for good measure.

While brushing should be primarily for grooming, not as a form of hair exercise, if you have dandruff, I think you should use your brush before shampooing in order to remove loose flakes gently.

Early in 1979 the National Cancer Institute released a report warning the public that selenium sulfide, an ingredient used in a 1 percent concentration in certain antidandruff shampoos, causes cancer in laboratory mice. The report further stated, however, that selenium sulfide is not normally absorbed through the scalp but can enter through open wounds. The maker of one of the shampoos containing this ingredient countered that the test findings had "little or no relationship to the human use of small quantities of this substance applied once or twice a week in a shampoo to the scalp for brief periods and then rinsed away." But what if you feel a need to shampoo four or five times a week? In that case, there are antidandruff shampoos that do not contain selenium sulfide, so check out labels before buying. You'll probably discover that after a certain period of time your antidandruff shampoo will appear to be less effective in controlling your dandruff. What's happened is that your scalp has built up an immunity to its dandruff-controlling properties, and that's your cue to switch brands. Eventually you'll probably be able to use your original shampoo again, and in most instances, it will work just fine.

HAIRCUT

Remember when woman wore hats? Back then I heard that when choosing a hat, Marlene Dietrich would have nothing to do with a hand-held mirror that focused solely on the face. Aware that while a hat was worn on the head, it was part of an overall look, she insisted on a full-length mirror. Well, the same principle applies to your haircut. You should take into account your physical proportions as well as the bone structure of your face and skull. The job of a good haircut, after all, is not only to make your hair look good but to make your *totality* look good, too, by giving balance to your facial features and to the relationship between your head and body.

Of course, you and your barber must also consider the texture of your hair. Fine or thinning hair can't be made to behave in the same accommodating way as medium- to coarse-textured hair that has more weight, and trying to make a few lank hairs behave and look as though they were many is a mistake. Fine or thinning hair should be worn fairly short and neat. Cutting close to the scalp will deemphasize the fact that you have less to comb. Furthermore, when worn short, hair like this has more body because it isn't being pulled down by added weight. How short you cut your hair depends on your facial features; not very short is the way to wear your hair if you have a prominent nose or large ears.

Happily, we've moved past the period when sideburns were worn so long that, as one wag put it, some men looked as though they could tuck theirs down into their undershorts. Some men who couldn't grow hair on their heads overcompensated by growing extravagant sideburns and threw their features out of balance as a result. Many a heavyset man with a round face, or a thin man with a narrow face, reasoned that the added hair would create the illusion of a narrower or broader face. Both were wrong. For some perverse reason, long sideburns make a round face look rounder, a thin face look even thinner. Fuller hair at the temples, however, does add the illusion of width to a narrow face.

If your hair's thin, you might consider getting a permanent. It not only adds body but also makes hair look thicker by changing the hair's chemical bonds. A permanent can sometimes be a boon, too, for a man with an oily scalp since perming lifts hair from the scalp and thus up and away from the overactive oil glands.

You might also consider one of the products now on the market that create the appearance of thicker hair by coating the hair shaft. A television commercial for one such product illustrates, figuratively, how it works. A model spreads the fingers of one hand wide to suggest how thin, separated hairs look and then simply brings her spread fingers together to suggest how hairs seem to grow together once the thickener is applied. It's only a temporary effect and washes out with the next shampoo, but it does work.

Women have always prized their hairdressers. Now the time has come for men to prize their barbers or, if you prefer, their hairstylists. Find one who considers a man's *totality* when he cuts his hair; avoid the old-timer who ties an apron around your neck and sees you as a disembodied head.

HAIR COLORING

Hair coloring has never been as good and as easy as it is now. Some men regard gray hair as a professional liability, and if you're one of them, don't hesitate to color your hair.

There are three basic kinds of hair coloring to consider: temporary, semipermanent, and permanent.

A *temporary* hair coloring is a rinse the color of which lasts only until your next shampoo. A rinse coats the outside of the hair shaft, has no effect on the structure of the hair, and, since it contains no bleaching agents, will make only a subtle change in the color of your hair. If your hair is graying, it won't take the gray away, but it will blend it in by adding a little color to it.

A *semipermanent* coloring also contains no bleaching agents, but unlike the temporary type, it not only coats the hair shaft but also penetrates its surface, with the result that it's more concentrated and makes a bigger color difference that lasts longer—usually through four or five shampoos.

A *permanent* hair coloring, on the other hand, lasts until your hair grows out or is cut because it not only penetrates the hair shaft but strips it as well to leave it more porous and the hair more receptive to a new color. A permanent coloring does cover the gray and does change the structure of hair because it contains a bleaching agent.

Should you have difficulty deciphering which products are temporary, semipermanent, and permanent, check for these clues usually found in the printed directions: "Lasts until it shampoos out" (temporary); "No peroxide"; "Lasts through three to five shampoos" (semipermanent); "Contains peroxide"; "Reapply every four to six weeks" (permanent).

When it comes to selecting a hair color (regardless of which of the three kinds you've decided to use), remember that the samples of color you see on charts and in the photos on the product boxes illustrate how the color will look on pure *white* hair. That color combined with that still in your hair will be a shade much darker than the one illustrated.

And while you may have had jet black hair or dark brown hair at twenty-five, at, say, fifty, you'd be making a big mistake if you were to color your hair that dark. Very dark hair looks dyed, and its severity also tends to flag attention to facial lines and any less than firm facial contours. Furthermore, chances are that your skin tone has changed as your hair grayed and that black or dark brown hair is no longer compatible with your complexion.

Of course, there are the metallic hair dyes, such as Grecian Formula 16 and Youthair, that contain a metal (usually lead or silver) which, when combed into the hair, coats it, reacting with the hair's protein to color the gray slowly over a period of several weeks. The effect isn't always as flattering as you might hope for, and sometimes the hair becomes brittle, though the dye really does no damage to the hair. Still, the value of these metallic dyes as a cover for gray is limited since they come only in dark colors and, as a result, are of little use to a man with light-colored hair.

Once you've chosen the kind of hair coloring in the specific shade you want, read the directions very carefully. You'll find that in most instances they call for two tests: a *patch* test for possible allergic reactions and a *strand* test to determine how the new shade works on your hair.

Here are a couple of rules to keep in mind once you've started coloring your hair:

1. Use a gentle shampoo specially created for hair color users because a harsh shampoo can remove the tint.
2. Avoid exposure to strong sunlight, which yellows colored hair.
3. After swimming, rinse out salt or chlorinated water at once.

If you have gray hair and are proud of it, make the most of it by using what's sometimes referred to as a gray hair enhancer. It will discourage a yellow tinge (certain medicated shampoos stain hair yellow). Clairol's Silk & Silver hair color lotion, sold in drug, food, and department stores, washes away yellow while adding silver highlights; it comes in a range of seven silvery shades, and each product box carries a photograph of a woman wearing the particular shade. The product advertising also features women, but don't let that put you off. Hair is hair, and has no gender, so go with the silvery shade of your choice.

BALDNESS:
How to Cope with It

The chief causes of baldness are threefold: age, the male hormone, and heredity. As we grow older, cells die and hair disappears from our scalps—often growing, instead, in our ears and nostrils. As women reach old age and their level of the female hormone (estrogen) drops, they lose hair, too (and often start growing facial hair), although baldness is much more prevalent among men because of the presence of the male hormone dihydrotesterone (DHT). Does that suggest that a bald man is more virile than a man with a full head of hair? No way. It's simply that one man will keep his hair because his follicles can survive despite the presence of the male hormone, while the man who goes bald can't, largely as the result of hereditary factors.

A man can inherit a tendency to baldness from either parent since a woman may also carry the hair-loss gene. While a woman's hair generally lasts 25 percent longer than a man's, if she carries the hair-loss gene and is given shots of male hormone, she, too, will start to lose hair. The bright side of this picture is that even in a family noted for its bald men, the inherited tendency to baldness can skip a generation.

Dr. Norman Orentreich, a leading New York dermatologist, believes that the key to checking hair loss before it starts may lie in blocking the effect of the male hormone. "Recent studies," he says, "have shown that it is possible to prevent androgenic DHT-induced hair loss without suppressing libido or potency. Steroids, such as progesterone, applied in tinctures or injected into the scalp, can safely reduce the production of DHT in the skin. And other steroids, not yet available in this country, offer further hope for safely arresting baldness." But all this is still in the testing stage. What can you do *now* to replace the hair you've already lost? A lot. Hair has its own built-in genetic clock, but you can pull the plug on yours.

The Hair Transplant

Senator William Proxmire has had a transplant, as have Frank Sinatra and television personality–writer Hugh Downs, not to mention hundreds of thousands of other men (and women) not in the public eye. The hair transplant is a form of minor surgery with a local anesthetic that, when done by a competent physician in his office, is completely safe and involves little or no discomfort. One doctor I visited has a portable TV set for his patients to watch while the surgery is being performed.

What happens is that grafts of hair are removed from the back and sides of the scalp (the so-called donor area) via a minute puncher and are then redistributed to the bald or balding areas. A totally bald man can't have a transplant for the obvious reason that there must be enough hair to be transplanted.

Since the 1950s this procedure has been generally accepted as the best and safest way to "grow" hair. The transplanted hair grows in with the same color, texture, and appearance as the hair where the grafts were taken. At each session some thirty to sixty transplants are usually done, the number of sessions depending on the number of transplants needed to restore a full head of hair. Each plug is a circular, cylindrical skin graft containing between fifteen and eighteen hairs which, after being transplanted, break off during the healing process. What remains in the scalp then are the healthy hair follicles, from which the newly transplanted hair, which should last a lifetime, begins to grow in about three months. It may require as few as 30 or 40 transplants to cover a slightly receding hairline or as many as 300 and upward for a more extensive area of baldness.

The cost is anywhere from $15 to $25 per plug, and it is estimated that the average man needs from 80 to 100 plugs.

Actually, there is another way of doing a transplant, and it's known as the flap technique. Here a strip of hair is lifted intact from along the side of the head behind the ear, with one end left attached so that it has blood vessels nourishing it, and is rotated at a ninety-degree angle up to a bald area. Developed by a Buenos Aires plastic surgeon, the flap technique is a three-stage operation, a major in-hospital procedure that, in the opinion of the majority of the doctors I spoke to, is fraught with problems. The transplanted hair, for example, grows in a backward direction, and the operation leaves a formidable scar. Still, one very respected plastic surgeon calls it "the future of natural-hair replacement," adding that it gives much thicker hair than can possibly be achieved with plugs alone.

The Hair Implant

Transplant and implant may sound similar, but the procedures (though both are minor surgery with a local anesthetic) are very different. Actually, the term "hair implantation" is a misnomer because no hair is *planted* anywhere. Basically it's simply a process to attach a custom-fitted hairpiece to your head permanently. Here's how it's done. Plastic or Teflon-coated wires are sutured into the scalp, and sections of these implants are left exposed on the patient's head to serve as anchors to which the hairpiece is attached. At the outset hair is cut from the patient's head so that the synthetic hair can be blended to match his natural color.

Unlike the hair transplant, the hair implant provides "instant hair," though not without a measure of discomfort and with the possibility of problems afterward. The anchors holding the hairpiece in place may become inflamed and infected, and in extreme cases, blood poisoning may occur. Furthermore, combing the hair is extremely difficult since the teeth of the comb can easily catch in the wire stitches.

The Hair Weave

This is a nonsurgical technique that weaves new hair, human or synthetic, strand by strand, into a porous webbing cut to the dimensions of the balding area; the new hair is then trimmed and styled to blend with the man's own hair. While hair weaving is, in my opinion, far superior to hair implantation, there are disadvantages to be considered. For instance, as the natural hair grows, the weave moves away from the scalp and so needs to be retightened in anywhere from four to ten weeks, meaning an added expense. Shampooing presents a problem, too, since it's necessary to wash beneath the weave or risk bacteria buildup and the unpleasant odor that accompanies it. The last but certainly not the least consideration is the fact that the weave must be replaced every two or three years as the hair wears out.

The Hairpiece

The hair in a hairpiece can be either human or synthetic. The synthetic costs less, lasts longer, but looks less attractive than real hair, which is harder to maintain and costs more, but it's well worth the extra money.

Since a hairpiece (nobody calls it a toupee anymore) is designed to cover a balding area rather than an entire head, it necessarily comes in different sizes and types.

The *hard top* has a plastic base with holes for ventilation into which the hairs are inserted. This type is the most durable because it has a hard base, but this also means it can be uncomfortable when worn in hot, humid weather.

The *soft top* has a base of soft mesh to which the hairs are tied. Not surprisingly, while this means the hairpiece is more comfortable to wear the year round, it doesn't have as long a life as the hard top.

The *mixed top* is exactly what its name suggests: a hairpiece that uses a soft mesh foundation near the edges and more solid foundation materials for the remainder of the hairpiece.

A hairpiece requires constant care. It should be brushed morning and night. If its hair is synthetic, shampoo the hairpiece no less than once a week to keep the hair loose; if its hair is natural, it can be cleaned by being submerged in a dry-cleaning solution. It goes without saying, I suppose, that after the hairpiece has been "dry-cleaned," it must be restyled.

At the start at least, it may take a man ten minutes or more to put his hairpiece on so that it looks natural and feels comfortable—and some of the soft tops, even some of the mixed tops, require an application of a little glue. One nice thing, though, is that unlike the case of the hair weave and hair implant, a man can take the hairpiece off and really wash his dome. A hairpiece should also be removed before one goes to bed or indulges in a strenuous sport since perspiration can affect the tape and, as a result, cause the piece to slip.

The life of a hairpiece is usually about three years.

The Wig

The job of a wig is to cover the entire dome, front to back. Here, too, the hair may be natural or synthetic. The natural tends to lose its color faster than the synthetic, but no matter what the origin of the hair used, a wig is less comfortable to wear in warm weather, and perspiration inevitably causes the hair to flatten. As far as care goes, a wig, like a hairpiece, must be brushed morning and night and should be cleaned no less than once a week. The man who wears a wig is advised to bring it back to where he bought it every couple of months to have it examined for any fiber loss and for reshaping.

Since a wig covers the whole top of the head, might it contribute to further loss of hair the man still has growing there? No, say the dermatologists.

For the man who is totally bald, there's no alternative other than to wear a wig or simply to face up to baldness, serene in the knowledge of what Yul Brynner and Telly Savalas have managed to accomplish with naked domes. And remember they *choose* to shave their skulls bare.

EXCESS BODY HAIR

Ironically, many a man has more hair on his body than he has on his head, and while a moderately hairy chest is usually considered macho, a hairy back isn't. In fact, when the hair on a man's chest takes on bushlike density, it's probably time he started pruning it; a pair of blunt-ended scissors will do the trick, trimming the chest hair just enough.

That works on the chest, but what about other parts of the anatomy? Tweezing or plucking breaks hair, and the only place for it is run-together eyebrows. Waxing, on the other hand, takes out the root. Women have been using the heated-wax technique on their legs for years. It can be done on any part of the body, and many skin care salons nowadays do it for men.

Electrolysis is the one proven way to remove unwanted hair permanently, but this is a fairly complicated procedure and should be done by a licensed electrologist. Depending upon the type of hair, its location, and its density, this procedure can sometimes require a sizable amount of time and money. But if superfluous body hair makes it embarrassing for you at the beach or poolside, by all means consider electrolysis.

For Clear, Firm Skin

Our skin is the largest organ of our bodies and has been described as "the shopping bag covering our other organs." Just keeping it clean isn't enough because your skin, after all, shows the first signs of aging. It requires intelligent care every day of your life.

Talking on the subject of skin care, one noted dermatologist said, "Don't smoke, don't drink, don't keep excessively late hours, don't sunbathe too much, and don't gain and lose weight constantly." Then, tongue in cheek, he added, "But first choose the right parents—ones with fairly oily olive skin." For while all skin dries as it ages, dry skin ages fastest.

In order to take proper care of your skin, you must know what type of skin you have. If you're not certain, here's a simple, foolproof test that will give you the answer:

1. Wash your face thoroughly, pat it dry with a towel, and wait thirty minutes.

2. Take three pieces of tissue, and mark them A, B, C.

3. Wipe Paper A over your forehead, Paper B over your nose, Paper C over each jaw.

4. If the tissue is unstained, your skin is dry in that area. Traces of oil mean your sebaceous glands are overactive. (One area where even a generally dry skin may show signs of oil is the nose.)

IF YOUR SKIN IS DRY

Choose a superfatted soap that cleans with a minimum of drying (all soaps are somewhat drying, removing the skin's oily top layer). After each washing or shaving, when your skin is still slightly damp, apply a moisturizer that will lubricate the outer layers of the skin and also work as a protective shield to hold in moisture. I think the New York dermatologist Dr. Richard Gibbs sums it up neatly when he says, "Skin dries out because it doesn't have enough water. Very simple." If that's the case, why can't you just use water to hydrate dry skin? Because you need something to *seal* the moisture in. Says Dr. Gibbs: "The protective shield provided by a moisturizer works sort of like wax paper around a sandwich." That is

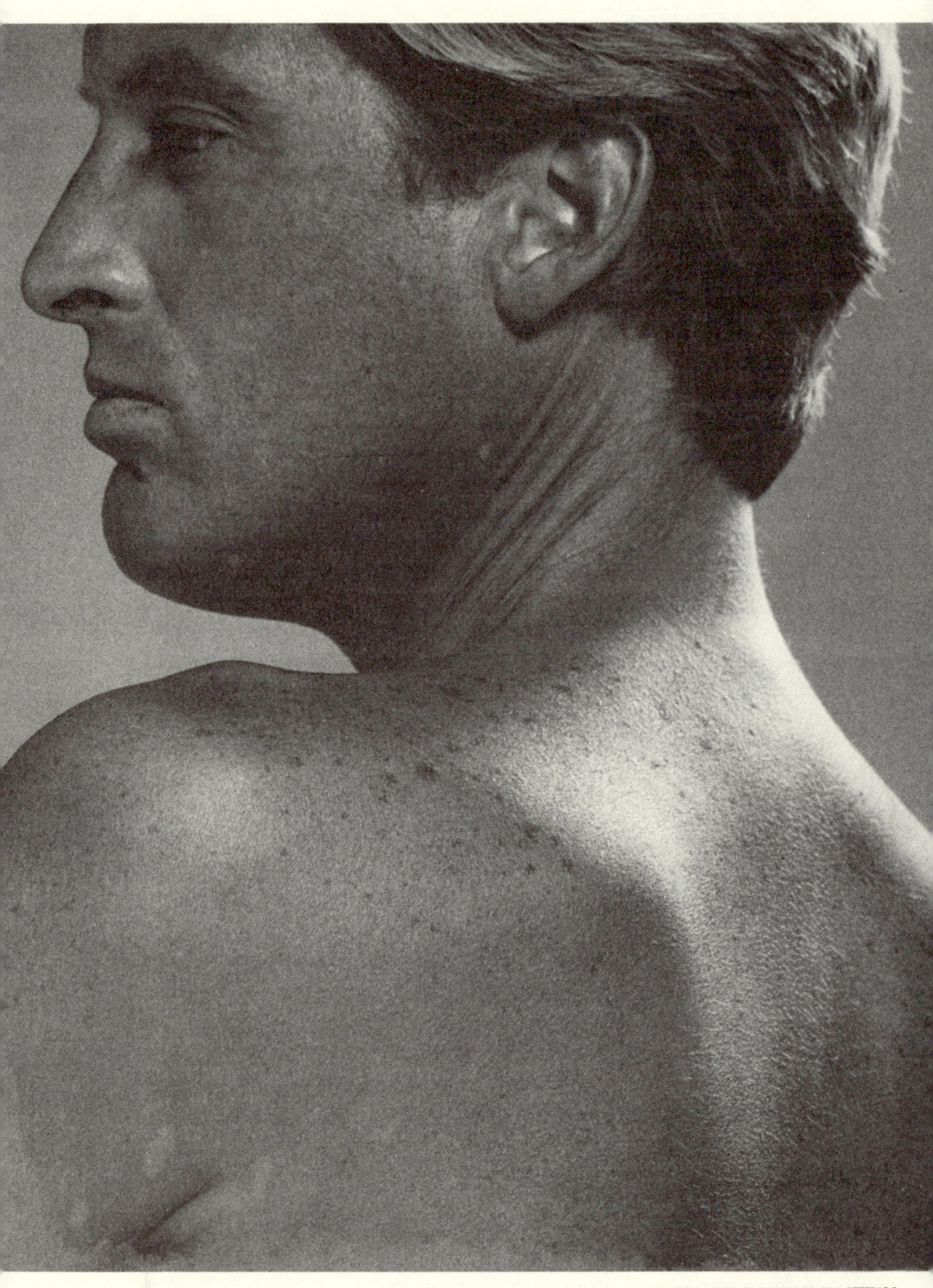

PHOTO BY ROBERT EPSTEIN.

why your moisturizer should be applied only to a freshly washed face, with some clear rinse water left on the dry areas.

But don't go overboard when it comes to using a moisturizer. During the humid summer months you perspire, and too much of a rich moisturizer can clog pores and even cause acnelike eruptions; in weather like that, you'd be wise to switch to a lighter product. And if your skin's dry only in certain areas, don't slather a moisturizer over your entire face; apply it just where it's needed.

You might try creating your own moisturizer. Recent experiments suggest that salt water can act as a moisturizing agent. Dr. Alexander Fisher, clinical professor of dermatology at the New York University Medical School, while treating men with chronically dry skin noted a marked improvement after salt-water swimming. In fact, two of his patients whose dry skin showed the most dramatic improvement had been swimming in the Dead Sea, noted for its high salt content. This has led Dr. Fisher to conclude that simple salinity, the presence of NaCl, hydrates the skin even better than store-bought moisturizers. (Swimming in chlorinated pool water has just the opposite effect.) So after washing your face clean, you might fill the basin with cool water, add a tablespoon of table salt, stir, and then splash it onto your dry skin areas.

Petroleum jelly also acts as a moisturizing agent. After washing your face, leave some clear rinse water on the dry areas, and smooth on some petroleum jelly to hold in the moisture.

Bath oil or foaming bath granules added to your bath water will also help you in the good fight against dehydration. Unfortunately much of the oil deposited on the skin during the bath is wiped off when drying with a towel afterward.

Oatmeal is a natural product recommended by many dermatologists for use in the tub when treating dry skin. Simply buy plain off-the-grocery-shelf oatmeal, and add about four to six tablespoons to your bath water.

The best advice I can give someone with dry skin is to rub himself all over with a body oil or just plain mineral oil immediately after he towels dry. And there's still another proven way to relieve dry skin: quick, lukewarm showers or baths. Too much soap and too hot water aggravate a dry skin condition.

So does indoor heating. When cold air is heated, it literally sucks moisture out of your skin. You can prove this by putting a pan of water on a radiator; the speed with which the water evaporates will show you just how much moisture is being sucked out of the air. The idea is to throw more moisture into the air, so invest in a humidifier or vaporizer, and leave it on until you go to sleep.

IF YOUR SKIN IS OILY

Use a detergent-based soap that will sop up excess oil that would otherwise clog pores and encourage blackheads. Between washings, put some witch hazel on a cotton ball or pad, and it will act like a blotter for oil. There are also some commercially prepared astringent pads you can carry in your pocket.

I suggest you treat your skin once a week to the extra-detergent action of cleansing grains, such as Clinique's Face Scrub, a tube of fine grains in a nongreasy base. Put a small amount in the palm of your hand, and then rub it into your wet skin, steering clear of the skin around your eyes; skin is thinnest there, and this rubbing action's too rugged for it. The cleansing grains will rub away not only excess oil but dead skin cells and grime in the bargain.

ROUGH SPOTS

There are sometimes areas on the body that look and feel parched —elbows, ankles, knees, for example. The solution is to remove the flaky layer of dead surface cells and get down to the fresh, moist cell layers underneath. It sounds like heavy going, but it isn't. A Buf-Puf is a nonmedicated cleansing sponge that works on the principle of epidermabrasion (*epiderm*=outer skin; *abrasion*=wearing away); you can take it into the tub or shower with you and gently buff away (the Buf Body Scrub with a long handle is specially designed for back and shoulders). Or you might try a pumice stone, which is an abrasive stone—actually volcanic lava that has cooled. Simply wet a piece, rub it with soap, and go over the rough spots with a circular motion. You can buy one in any drugstore.

Since I don't know of any skin that isn't in need of some lubrication after a tub or shower, I suggest you rub yourself all over with a body oil after toweling dry. If your skin tends to be oily, pat on some talc to blot any excess oil.

THE RAZOR BLADE versus THE ELECTRIC RAZOR

Dr. Norman Orentreich, one of America's most widely quoted dermatologists, believes most men shave poorly because they try to scrape away the beard in a kind of one-step maneuver. A good barber, he points out, "lathers, shaves . . . lathers, shaves . . . lathers, shaves. He never tries to do a thorough shave with one lathering." In short, what the barber is doing each time is softening the top layers of the skin and that way making it possible for the razor blade to *glide* over the skin. Result: a great shave that has a rejuvenating effect on the skin.

Every time you shave you're shaving off not only your beard but the top layer of skin as well. You are, in a sense, creating new and vital skin. For that reason I personally opt for a razor blade shave in preference to one with an electric razor. "Cold-knife shaving" is what Dr. Orentreich calls it. "I don't care what kind of blade it is—single-edge, double-edge, whatever. . . . But for the cleanest shave and the best-looking skin, I like a razor blade, a sharp knife, cold steel. . . . When a man shaves with lather and a blade razor, his skin looks younger, too."

As for an after-shave lotion, if you have dry skin, avoid the perfumed variety because they're drying; a splash of cold water will do just fine. If you have oily skin, you might try witch hazel.

FACIAL MASKS

Women have used them for centuries. The very earliest ones were of clay, but today there are masks for men which can be divided into two categories: the *rinse-off* and *peel-off* kinds. Both kinds are applied only to a freshly cleansed face.

Dermatologists aren't exactly enthusiastic about masks and the claims made for them: that they create a younger appearance, help eliminate wrinkles, deep-clean pores (nobody knows what "deep-clean" means), and moisturize the skin. What do masks *really* do? Well, since most of them shrink as they dry, they appear to give facial lines a temporary ironing, while revving up circulation and thereby giving skin a pleasant glow. The benefits are temporary—an hour or two at best—but this isn't to say that masks are of no value. A mask is literally a facial treatment—nothing more, nothing less. And you do look better—fresher, more rested—and that's no little improvement.

Should you decide to try a mask, you have a king-sized collection to choose from. There are cleansing masks that are especially good for oily skin since they contain abrasives that do a pretty thorough

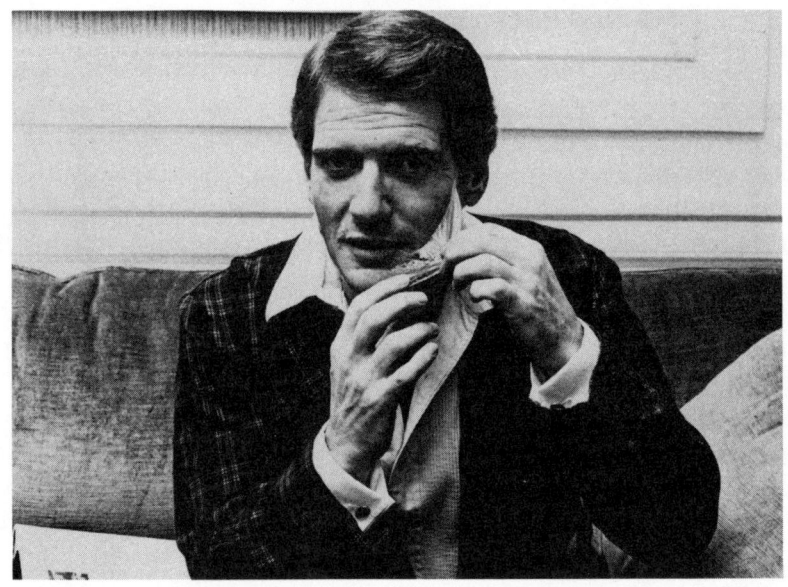

A facial mask of the peel-off variety. PHOTO COURTESY OF MEN'S FASHION ASSOCIATION.

cleaning job, and there are moisturizing masks that give aid to dry, thirsty skin. Both the peel-off masks and the gel masks that rinse off with water are mild enough to be good for almost any type of skin.

You can, if you wish, make your own mask. A honey-and-egg mask is recommended for dry skin. All you have to do is take a tablespoon of strained honey and one egg yolk (egg white is drying), and beat together with a fork or, better yet, an egg beater if there's one handy. Apply the mixture to your face (neck, too, if you like), let it remain on for fifteen minutes, and remove the mask with a soft towel dipped in lukewarm water.

An oatmeal mask is a paste of dry oatmeal and warm water, and it's a better-than-average degreaser for oily skin. Pat it on, and as soon as it's dry, rinse it off with clear, cold water.

Warning: If you use a make-it-yourself mask, don't put any food on your face to which you're usually allergic.

Never apply any facial mask, commercial or homemade, around the eyes, mouth, or nostrils. Masks can be extremely difficult to remove from areas other than skin itself.

Never leave a mask on overnight; they're to be removed *completely* when they've done their job. Peel-off masks aren't rinsed, but pulled off, but if any residue remains behind, rinse it off.

THE FACIAL

As far as I'm concerned, the most important thing about a facial is the fact that it cleanses the skin and soothes the psyche. What with pollution today, maintaining a really clean skin isn't all that easy, and as for the psyche, there's something about being the focal point of someone's undivided attention for, say, a half hour or so—their sensitive fingertips having a go at your skin—that's tantamount to a short vacation. By the time your facial is over you feel so relaxed that even if you didn't look all that different, you'd look at your reflection in the mirror and tell yourself you did. But the nice thing is that when a facial is done properly, you actually do look better. Furthermore, the results are longer-lasting than those of a facial mask.

I make a point of saying when a facial is done *properly*, for the very good reason that if your skin isn't in the hands of a thoroughly trained and knowledgeable individual, a facial can be harmful—stretching the skin via pulling and tugging. Skin stretches with time, and that is how flaps, folds, and pouches form. You don't have to pay to have someone do that for you.

You can go to a barber and get yourself what's known as a salon facial, or you can go to a dermatologist for what's known as a medical facial, the difference being that a dermatologist is, by virtue of his training, much more knowledgeable about skin care than a barber. Still, there are men I know who prefer the salon facial, which is usually somewhat less expensive, and they argue, unless you have a skin problem, why spend the extra dollars?

A friend of mine goes every couple of weeks to a salon for a one-hour facial given by a titian-haired lady with a Liverpool accent and a framed photograph of Queen Elizabeth on the wall. She's been giving facials since 1951 and says that about half her customers nowadays are men. I watched as my friend stripped to the waist and settled back in a barbershop type of chair, and she draped a towel across his chest.

"He has very fine-texture skin that needs loads and loads of cream," she said, beginning to massage a rich lanolin-based cream laced with almond oil into his face and back, after which she applied a muslin cloth dampened with an all-purpose cleansing lotion. "Now this is like a *deep* cleanser," she explained as she proceeded to paint on a medicated lotion with a small brush. As the lotion dried, she lathered on still more of the original cream, her fingers kneading the flesh of his neck and shoulders. Then, after applying more of the cream to his face with a brush, she very gently worked it into the areas around his eyes and mouth. If she hadn't kept up a steady stream of conversation, I wager he'd have fallen asleep at this point.

Having cranked the chair into a perfectly horizontal position, she started massaging him from the chin clear down to the base of his throat. Only then did she begin massaging the skin on his face. "This keeps the facial muscles in good form," she said. "You've got to do everything you can to help nature. Most of us don't understand the importance of starting young." She nodded in the direction of the photograph on the wall. "Queen Elizabeth started getting facials at sixteen."

She applied more cream, after which she started kneading his skin with a wider upward and circular motion. She pressed a damp muslin cloth onto his face ("to get all the goo off") and then washed it with a super-fatted soap made for dry skin. Next, having covered his eyes with pads, she concluded by spraying his face and neck with what she called "a finishing lotion to close the pores." The cost of this one-hour treatment: $25 and a $5 tip. The result: My friend's skin looked clear and refreshed, and he certainly felt far more relaxed than he had an hour earlier.

The next day I visited the spacious offices of a dermatologist where medical facials are given by a licensed beautician who formerly worked at a Fifth Avenue beauty salon. What makes this a *medical* facial? The doctor examines the skin beforehand and instructs what products are to be used. "Your dermatologist is the only professional person who can totally analyze your skin for precancerous lesions, seborrhea, dermatitis, acne, and other skin conditions," I was told. "Laymen in this field may sometimes cause more harm than good." A tiny white wart, for example, might spread if a routine facial were given. And a dermatologist will advise creams be used only if the skin happens to be extremely dry.

This particular medical facial starts with a cleansing of the skin with a soap, after which the face is steamed ("a very light steam") to soften the sebum so that blackheads and whiteheads can be removed. In a salon facial, it was explained, blackheads and whiteheads are almost always removed with fingernails wrapped in a paper handkerchief. At the doctor's office an extremely small instrument is used, after which a white-of-egg mask is applied to soothe the skin. Once the mask dries, it is removed with a natural sponge. Finally, according to the skin's particular needs, either a moisturizing lotion (dry skin) or a powder-based lotion (oily skin) is applied.

A medical facial usually costs anywhere from $30 to $35, and I was told that "people who live in city areas should have a facial once every four to six weeks to protect the skin from pollution."

CAMOUFLAGE

Touchup, makeup—call it what you will. The idea behind these flesh-colored sticks is to conceal tiny flaws, shadows, dark circles under the eyes, and lines. Some come in a range of shades; others offer one shade which somehow manages to blend in with your skin tone. Packaged in a case like a lipstick, it is applied directly to the skin or dabbed on your fingertip first and then applied to the skin with the fingertip.

A little bit of mineral oil in the formula prevents any drying or caking. From what I've been able to observe, these concealing sticks are most effective in playing down ("concealing," I think, puts it a bit too strongly) lines under the eyes and the nasal-labial fold—the deep line from the side of the nose to the side of the mouth. Some men I know who would ordinarily never think of using one of these sticks never fail to use one when having a business portrait taken. The combination of the photographer's strong lights and the softening effects of the stick sometimes will erase as many as five to ten years from a man's appearance.

A SUNTAN WITH NONE OF THE RISK

That's what a moisturizing skin bronzer can do for you. Its product formula contains purified water, which is what makes it a *moisturizing* bronzer. Still, I advise that you apply yours to a damp (not altogether wet, just slightly damp) skin and thereby assure that the bronzer will go on smoothly, soften your skin, and stay moist longer. It goes without saying, I suppose, that a bronzer goes on a freshly cleansed face.

Some bronzers are put out in a selection of shades, but nowadays more are in just one medium shade, and that way the more you apply, the darker your skin will look. Since a natural suntan should be acquired gradually, let that be a guide to the sly way you should use your bronzer; let your color subtly deepen over a period of time.

Some bronzers come in the form of a gel; others are in a solid stick form, which you can rub directly on your face. I'm partial to the gel for a couple of reasons. I prefer squeezing the gel onto my fingertips and then blending it in with my fingers; the stick, on the other hand, seems to me tantamount to rubbing a bar of dark soap on my face, and it feels drying, although I realize that this is an illusion. But no two ways about it, a gel in a tube is far more packable than a stick and travels more easily.

If your bronzer doesn't contain a moisturizer and you have dry skin, by all means use a moisturizer under your bronzer. If you're using a concealing stick for camouflage, use it before applying your bronzer. If you're using both a moisturizer *and* a concealing stick, no problem: first, the concealing stick, then the moisturizer, and finally, the bronzer.

Unless you use your bronzer very lightly—just enough to give your face a faint glow—you'd best apply some to your neck, too, front and back. If you've ever seen a man with a bronzed face and the back of his neck the color of a fish belly, you know how comical it looks. Apply your bronzer to your neck before you put your shirt on; if not, tuck some tissue in the neck of your shirt to avoid staining it.

What about your hands? You can forget your palms, but if you're choosing to give your face a fairly deep bronze shade, you must apply some of the bronzer to the backs of your hands. Avoid your fingers and knuckles, though; the creases there simply won't take kindly to the added color, which will settle in and look about as attractive as, say, a line of grime under a fingernail. While we're on the subject of a bronzer and your hands, note that they stain when you apply a gel. No worry, however. Simply wash the color off with soap and warm water. But bear in mind that a bronzer is quick-drying (one of its *plus* factors), so wash your hands as soon as you've finished applying the bronzer.

BLOCK THAT SUN!

Dr. Cyril Marsh, New York dermatologist, estimates that perhaps better than 50 percent of the aging that occurs to skin (drying, wrinkling, loss of elasticity) is due to the sun, and overexposure to the sun is every bit as damaging to a man's skin as it is to a woman's. But in the opinion of Suzy Chaffee, Olympic skier, men are the worst when it comes to protecting themselves from the sun. "I don't know if it's from a sense of machismo or whether they're simply unaware of the consequences," she says, "but I've seen guys seemingly age five years only one year after taking up outdoor sports—simply because they didn't bother to apply a suntan lotion."

Dr. Bedford Shelmire, Jr., in his book *The Art of Looking Younger* (St. Martin's Press, 1973), puts it this way: "A few months of intense sun exposure can produce more aging changes than a century of normal wear." Aging skin is only part of the story. "Lying around under the sun is the worst thing you can do to your skin. It's the single greatest cause of prematurely aging skin, and can lead to skin cancer," warns Dr. Stephen Kurtin, a dermatologist who teaches at Mount Sinai Hospital in New York. Skin cancer is directly related to the degree of exposure to the sun, and there are more cases occurring in the states below the Mason-Dixon line, where there's more sunshine, than elsewhere.

Yet few of us want to avoid the sunshine altogether. A handsome tan can be a morale booster, a tonic for the personality. Fortunately precautions against sun damage are simple. There are basically two kinds of preparations that offer protection.

Sunscreens—liquids or creams—filter out those ultraviolet rays that burn (UVB rays) but allow you to tan from the less harmful rays (UVA rays). Read the label, and see to it that yours contains at least 5 percent PABA (para-aminobenzoic acid), which is the best chemical screening agent money can buy. For people who are allergic to PABA, there are other good chemical screens that include pdimethylaminobenzoate, cinnamates, phenyl, and benzophenones.

Sunblocks, not to be confused with sun lotions, prevent *all* rays from getting through and, as a result, prevent tanning as well as burning. They wash off in the water and must be reapplied.

Now there are suntanning products that contain no sunscreens. Many of these contain coconut or other oils and are, actually, nothing more or less than skin moisturizers, offering no protection against burning; that explains why their labels most often read that they're made for those who "tan easily."

Even when you've slathered yourself with the most effective sunscreen product, there are certain rules to remember. "Sun, like food, should be taken in moderation," is the way Dr. Albert Lefkovitz, a leading New York dermatologist, puts it.

Your first day's exposure should be limited to twenty minutes maximum. If you have fair skin, I'd say pare that first day's exposure down to ten to fifteen minutes. Then, no matter what your skin type, add no more than five minutes to your time in the sun for the next five days, at which time a new pigment should start to darken your skin, and by the week's end you should have enough to protect yourself from burning.

Sun's rays are their most intense between eleven in the morning and three in the afternoon. Also, be aware that you needn't stretch out in the sunshine to get a burn; sunlight bounces off water and sand so that you're not entirely safe even when sitting beneath a wide beach umbrella.

On overcast, foggy days it's possible to get a sunburn, and even snow reflects the sun's burning rays—as much as 85 percent. So whenever and wherever you're exposed to sunshine—summer or winter—play it safe, and protect your skin. And remember, your hands are always exposed; you can't often wear gloves while playing sports, but you can—and should—use a sunscreen or a sunblock.

Keep using your sunscreen even after you've developed a good tan. The protection it provides washes off with each swim, with perspiration, so it must be reapplied. In fact, I suggest you make it a rule to reapply yours every two hours even if you've done nothing more active than shifted position in your chair.

It's also wise when you take the sun to steer clear of using scented preparations which may contain an oil that might cause adverse reactions when the skin is exposed to the sun.

A sunlamp in place of the sun? Why bother now that there are skin bronzers to be had and especially when exposure to artificial sunlight poses about as much threat to skin as real sunlight since both forms of sunlight give off ultraviolet rays?

I grew up hearing about the fast-tanning effects of oil (baby or mineral) mixed with iodine. Well, neither oil when applied to the skin offers protection from the sun's rays, and iodine adds nothing more than a film of stain. Too thick an application of oil can clog pores, and when you add perspiration, you can end up with an itchy rash. In short, mineral or baby oil mixed with iodine neither prevents sunburn nor promotes a suntan.

Now what if, despite every precaution, you somehow manage to get a burn? The best you can hope for is a slight temporary relief. The more uncomfortable areas may be covered with cool, wet compresses, and a moisturizing cream or lotion will soothe as well as relieve dryness. Most important of all, stay out of the sun until the symptoms disappear. Unfortunately the tanning process occurs much more gradually than the burning process, so let common sense and moderation prevail.

Meanwhile, there's good news in that the Food and Drug Administration has recently established standards that will tell you exactly the degree of protection you can expect from a sunscreen or sunblock. The rating system will be based on a scale of 2 to 15. If a product has a sun protection factor of, say, 2, that means you can stay in the sun for twice as long as you could if you had no protection at all. So a safe ten-minute exposure becomes twenty minutes long when you use an SPF-2 rated product; SPF-3 stretches it to thirty minutes, and so on.

Still another happy note: According to Dr. Irwin I. Lubowe, dermatologist, people react differently to the sun according to their ages. Men are most vulnerable to sunburn between the ages of thirty and thirty-five and most resistant to sunburn between the ages of fifty and sixty.

PLASTIC SURGERY

What's the point in feeling young if you don't *look* young? That's apparently the way a lot of men are figuring these days. Plastic surgery—call it cosmetic or aesthetic or corrective surgery, if you want to—is the answer for an increasing number of them in their forties, fifties, sixties, even seventies, who want to erase the worrisome wrinkles, sagging jowls, and eye bags of advancing age. "The knife" can change not only a man's outer appearance but often his personality and outlook on life as well.

What ages a man? Dr. Laurence R. LeWinn, assistant professor of surgery at the New York Hospital–Cornell Medical Center, says: "I put a lot of emphasis on a man's genetic makeup." A plastic surgeon in Southern California who estimates that more than half his patients today are men, answers the same question: "It's a combination of heredity, plus physical, personality types and temperament." Most of his patients, he adds, see a younger-looking face as a decided advantage in the competition with younger men in business.

One of the country's most eminent plastic surgeons describes cosmetic surgery as different from any other surgery in that "it is not really necessary for health and survival. It is elective and selective—elective in the sense that the patient elects to have it done and that the doctor elects to accept doing the procedure for the patient and selective in the sense that the patient can select that portion of the anatomy which he would like corrected."

"What men are most concerned about," says Dr. LeWinn, "is any sign of aging that makes them look tired or as if they were slowing down. Years have nothing to do with it; men, as a rule, don't mind some lines in their faces—they feel this gives character. It's the appearance of being old and worn down that they want to get rid of. Here they are, functioning very well, but they worry about being considered over the hill."

The Face-Lift

Quite often there's one particular moment when a man decides to have a face-lift. A Dallas businessman in his mid-sixties recalls that moment: "I walked by a department-store window mirror one day and asked myself, 'Who's that old man with the styled hair?'" He decided then and there that he wasn't going "to continue wearing puffs under my eyes and bulges under my chin."

A friend of mine, also in his mid-sixties, said he decided to have surgery when he looked at an old passport photo of himself with something resembling admiration—"and when it was taken ten years ago, I thought I looked a mess." He had a face-lift, and now, seven years later, he's planning to have the operation again. "I never intend to grow old until I feel old!" he says.

Two face-lifts. How many times can a man undergo the operation? "There's almost no limit," says Dr. LeWinn, "but two is the usual limit." If that sounds somewhat contradictory, so be it. Although he's a plastic surgeon married to a plastic surgeon, Dr. LeWinn makes a point of cautioning men about the "biological price" they may have to pay for facial surgery. For starters, the operation leaves scars on the scalp—a problem if a man is bald. Warns another plastic surgeon: "A man may find his sideburns growing a lot closer to the front of his ears," and in a few cases the sideburns have been eliminated altogether. Still another problem is that a beard area now extends behind the ears onto the neck; that, says Dr. LeWinn, "means a man has to be willing to shave behind his ears, and some men object to the idea. In fact, if a man is heavily bearded, this may rule him out as a candidate for a face-lift."

Still, a successful face-lift can often make a profound change in a man's life, and no longer is such an operation considered an act of pure narcissism. A man having cosmetic surgery today can take comfort in the fact that it's now considered psychologically healthy to want to look one's best.

But face it, a face-lift is more than a tuck here and a tuck there. Most surgeons arrange for pictures of the patient before surgery to serve as a guide during the operation; the pictures are taken by a professional photographer in a strong and in no way flattering light. The object, after all, says Dr. LeWinn, "is to show certain standard views that help the surgeon—front view, side view to see jowls, sagging eyelids, etc." Eyelid surgery is often done in conjunction with the face-lift.

The patient usually checks into the hospital the day before the operation, at which time tests are done on blood, blood pressure, urine, heart, and lungs. The patient is told to abstain from taking aspirin for two weeks before the operation since the chronic use of aspirin can slow down the blood's capacity to clot.

A face-lift (rhytidectomy) is major surgery that can take anywhere from three to five hours. It may be done under local or general anesthesia. If a local is used, preoperative sedatives are administered, beginning the evening before. If a general anesthesia is used, the patient is instructed not to eat or drink for eight hours before surgery. Briefly, the operation consists of strategically planned incisions which allow the surgeon to correct the aging areas by pulling up the skin and drawing the subcutaneous tissue into place. Small scars are thus buried in areas where they'll not be seen: behind the ears, in temple hairlines, or in normal skin folds. The redraping of the skin is the crucial point in the operation, for it's then that the surgeon determines just how tight to pull the skin and just how much to cut away.

A large bandage wrapped around the patient's head performs three functions: It (1) supports tissues; (2) stops bleeding under the tissues; and (3) minimizes postoperative swelling. The bandage remains on for anywhere from one to two days after surgery. The sutures that show in the front of the ears and around the eyelids are usually removed on the fifth day after surgery, and the remaining sutures—mostly in the hairline—are finally removed about two and a half weeks after surgery. By the time all sutures are out, there's usually only a trace of bruising and puffiness, and the patient's face starts to get the look he had the operation for.

Most face-lifts prove effective for five to eight years. The younger the man, the better his chances for long-lasting results. The cost? At this writing it's in the neighborhood of $2,500 plus hospital expenses. Actually there's no such thing as a standard fee; what determines the cost is the city in which the surgery is performed and the reputation of the surgeon.

Now a word about the "fifteen-minute tuck," as it's sometimes called. What it is is an abbreviated face-lift that, despite the fifteen-minute tag, actually requires an hour and supposedly stays put for two or, maybe, three years. I've never known anyone who has admitted to having one, so I can't attest to its success. Suffice to say that when I attempted to interview one plastic surgeon who has made a certain reputation (and gained a fair amount of press) via the facial tuck operations performed in his office with local anesthesia, I was told he no longer granted interviews.

Although an abbreviated face-lift costs a fraction of a bona fide face-lift, I tend to equate it with, say, a fast-food chain versus a gourmet restaurant. You get what you pay for. Perhaps it's the use of the diminutive "tuck" that bothers me. A knife is a knife, and when it cuts into the skin, that's surgery. I can't go along with the newspaper scribe who regards the "fifteen-minute tuck" as the first step toward turning cosmetic surgery "into a part of the average routine, like a trip to the dentist." No way.

Chemabrasion—chemical face peeling—is often used for conditions for which a face-lift isn't effective: horizontal lines on the forehead, fine vertical lines on the upper lip ("prune lip"), and wrinkling around the eyes. Sometimes, in fact, during the face-lift operation a chemical peel may be done to such areas of the face. Carbolic acid is the chemical most frequently used.

No anesthesia is used, but the patient is premedicated so that he's thoroughly relaxed, and if only a small area of the face is going to be peeled, the operation may be done in the doctor's office rather than in a hospital. As the chemical solution is applied to the face, the skin instantly turns a frosty white and then, in a matter of minutes, becomes swollen and turns dark red. What's happening is that the chemical solution is eating away the outer layer and part of the inner layer of the skin—a second-degree burn is the result— thus stimulating new skin growth. Scabs form, and when they separate within a week or ten days, the new skin is smoother, firmer, and smaller-pored than the old. Nevertheless, because the new skin will gradually age, results of a peeling are certainly not permanent. Still, the process can be repeated again in another year or two if thought necessary.

This is considered surgery (superficial chemosurgery), and it must be done by a dermatologist or plastic surgeon. The American Medical Association condemns its practice by nonmedical personnel.

Dermabrasion—surgical planing—is a *smoothing* operation to eradicate light wrinkles, fine lines, and the pits and scars that are the residue of severe acne. The outer layers of the skin are scraped with a motor-driven dermabrader that works rather like a dentist's high-speed drill. Depending on how deep a planing is necessary, a variety of sizes and textures of wire brushes may be attached to the dermabrader, and the depth of the planing may also determine where the operation is performed (doctor's office or hospital) and whether a general anesthesia is used or whether a skin refrigerant (usually ethyl chloride) is simply sprayed over the area being treated to freeze out the pain.

As with chemical peeling, the face is treated in sections, and a full-face treatment is carried into the hairline and just below the jawline so that there will be no difference in pigmentation color between the planed and unplaned sections. Scabs form and separate in seven to ten days, although a pinkish surface usually requires another three or four weeks to fade completely.

Silicone injections are generally considered the best method of treating wrinkles—that is, liquid silicone that has been filtered, purified, and sterilized. Used judiciously in very small amounts, this medical grade of silicone can produce excellent results.

Dr. Robert Auerbach of the New York University College of Medicine says, "I have a sneaking suspicion that we are doing almost as many men with wrinkles as women." He reports that men mainly want the nasal-labial fold—the deep line running from the side of the nose to the side of the mouth—made less prominent, although pure liquid silicone is also being increasingly used to soften forehead lines and lines between the eyebrows.

Dermatologists have been using silicone, first discovered in 1943, since about 1967. It's a compound derived from silica (quartz), which is what one-quarter of the earth is made of. The medical grade of fluid silicone has the consistency of mineral oil and can be injected into any depressed area of the face with a thirty-gauge needle—the finest needle made—a fifth of a drop at a time. As each droplet penetrates beneath the deepest stratum of the skin, it's surrounded by a lacing of fibrous tissues that keeps it in place. The injections feel like tiny pinpricks, and after they have been given, the patient is asked to press firmly over the area to prevent black-and-blue marks.

The doctor's expertise comes into play when he determines the number of droplets to be injected at each session. The area of the face being treated builds up gradually, so this is a multiple-injection technique that usually takes place over a period of several months, the injections given at intervals roughly a month apart. Dr. Orentreich, quoted earlier, was one of the first dermatologists asked to study liquid silicone skin injections clinically and report on their progress to the federal Food and Drug Administration; he describes liquid silicone injections as "a controlled way of building skin." Today only a small number of doctors have access to medical-grade silicone; for the name of a physician in your area who uses liquid silicone therapy, write the American Society of Plastic and Reconstructive Surgeons, Inc., 29 East Madison Street, Chicago, Illinois 60602.

COSMETIC ACUPUNCTURE

This has been described in some circles as a face-lift that involves no stitches, swelling, discoloration, or pain—in short, a face-lift without surgery. This is not totally accurate, and people who are directly involved avoid saying so, although they do claim that this ancient Chinese needle art can remove years from the face and they refer to it as a process of rejuvenation and revitalization.

Dr. Ralph Sepson at the Acupuncture Treatment Center in New York City says, "We don't know how it works. Patients think something happens. Something does happen."

What specifically? Well, the center has treated more than 1,000 men and women with cosmetic acupuncture and concedes that it works with some and not with others. The center's literature says, "It may erase as many as five to fifteen years from any face, with results apparent after just a few treatments. Fine lines may be entirely erased. Deep-set lines may be reduced while bags around the neck and eyes may be firmed." But Dr. Sepson cautions, "You have to suspend your Western way of thinking. Explaining acupuncture is trying to impose a logic on top of something you know works. There's really no scientific understanding of what it does."

All this might not sound very convincing except for the fact that acupuncture has survived as a science-art-philosophy for about 5,000 years, and I think we all know proved stories of Westerners who have come back from China cured of a longtime ailment via the strategically placed needles of an acupuncturist when years of medical treatment here in the States had failed.

Even more intriguing is the fact that the fine-as-a-hair needle, which makes even the slender one used for silicone injections seem large, may be inserted nowhere near, say, a sag, jowl, or wrinkled eyelid that's being treated. As one acupuncturist explains, "We stimulate the appropriate nerve with the needles, which causes a contraction, tightening up the facial muscles, and in so doing lifts." Another acupuncturist says that the needles stimulate blood circulation to the face, which tightens up the muscle tone, fills out hollows, and helps stave off the dryness that leads to wrinkles. Furthermore, with acupuncture a man can come back to it as needed, taking booster treatments whenever he wants them.

The length of each treatment seems to depend on the condition of the skin. Needles may remain in place anywhere from twenty to forty minutes, and most acupuncturists agree that there has to be a minimum of seven sessions before a patient sees results. How long will the rejuvenated look last? Apparently anywhere from two to five years, and whether that means booster treatments along the way I don't know. Frankly, I don't think that this suggests elusiveness on the part of the acupuncturists so much as the fact that, as Dr. Sepson says, even they don't know how it works or why it works well for some and not for others. Some people, for example, who have gone to an acupuncturist to keep arthritis under control have found that they were getting an extra bonus: Their faces were looking firmer, younger.

Don't get the idea, however, that cosmetic acupuncture is a matter of lying back and being stuck with a few needles. What makes this a science-art-philosophy is the acupuncturist's expertise in what shape needle to use, the angle at which it should be inserted, and how long it should stay in.

The price for all this is minor compared to the cost of a surgical face-lift. Each session usually runs anywhere from $25 to $35, although there's no way of anticipating how many sessions a man will require before seeing results. It would seem that he should expect an investment of somewhere between $500 and $1,000. Sounds almost like a bargain, doesn't it? But remember that even the acupuncturist can't promise that you'll be one of the people who'll see results. Still, cosmetic acupuncture is a fascinating subject, and there are increasing numbers of people who regard it as the newest way to stay young-looking longer.

CELL THERAPY

It's a needle again, but this time it's a hypodermic needle injecting live cells of sheep fetuses. This therapy is based on the premise that the death of the body's cells accelerates the aging process. Or to be more exact, when the rate of reproduction of new cells falls below the rate of dying cells, we're in trouble.

The cell therapists contend that injecting these live cells into the body (from sheep because of their resistance to disease) stimulates cell growth and rejuvenates it. The American Medical Association doesn't agree, and as a result, cell therapy isn't practiced in the United States—yet. In fact, fresh-cell therapy isn't practiced outside Switzerland, where it came into prominence back in 1931. Professor Paul Niehans, the high priest of cell therapy, died in 1975 at age eighty-four, but his work is still going on at the Clinic La Prairie in Clarens, where the treatment takes one week and costs in the neighborhood of $3,000. One hears that everyone from Winston Churchill and Charles de Gaulle to Charlie Chaplin and the Duke and Duchess of Windsor has been a patient at the clinic, but nobody knows for sure. What we do know, however, is that Niehans did treat Pope Pius XII in 1954 when he was seventy-seven and dangerously ill, and the Pontiff recovered and credited the fresh-cell injections.

Early in 1979 the Clinic La Prairie introduced a five-product line of facial creams and a body lotion made in the clinic. Available in a handful of stores in this country, the five products sell for a hefty $235, but it's possible to buy the products separately (the body lotion, for example, sells for $40).

Peter Stephan is in his thirties, and that makes him the youngest of the so-called youth doctors, although he's not a doctor. He is the very affluent proprietor of the Cell Therapy Center, located in a posh London town house, where I interviewed him some years ago.

It was his father, a physician, who, in the 1950s, introduced cell therapy—with certain variations—into Britain. Young Stephan calls his treatment body servicing. A typical treatment involves four injections at each of five sessions, two shots in each buttock each time. The cost is slightly under $1,000 (you don't stay at the center), and Stephan told me that he treats an average of 1,000 new patients yearly, including members of the House of Lords.

When I talked to him, Stephan bridled somewhat at the notion that cell therapy is reserved only for the old. "It's valuable for people of all ages," he insisted. "It's much easier for the cell therapists to avoid symptoms of aging than it is to alleviate them once they're present." Granting that one can't turn the clock back and become young again, he still stated: "However, the results of cell therapy are often very startling. When a patient returns for examination after treatment it's found that the entire system has undergone a mental and physical overhaul. The patient is much more alert and has more energy. His figure improves, and the whole outlook changes beneficially."

H-3

Dr. Ana Aslan runs the seventy-four-acre Geriatrics Institute in Bucharest, Romania, and her wonder drug Gerovital (essentially procaine, more commonly called novocaine, plus benzoic acid and metasulfide of potassium), discovered by her in 1957, has prompted Nobel Laureate Miguel Angel Asturias to proclaim publicly: "Madame Aslan's medicine has given me back the pleasure of living and the supreme joy of creating."

A former cardiologist, Dr. Aslan is nearly eighty, and according to a friend of mine who has been a patient at the clinic, she has the smooth skin of a woman half her age. Treated with H-3, which is said to revitalize dormant cells, some of her patients have supposedly grown new hair and others' gray hair has returned to its natural color. The first two weeks of injections—along with physiotherapy, special diet, and mineral waters—are given at the clinic, and then the patient is given a one-year treatment program to continue when he returns home. The clinic claims that no results can be expected before three months.

Compared to cell therapy, this treatment is relatively inexpensive. In fact, the Romanian National Tourist Office in New York City now has a two-week all-expense tour that includes airfare from New York City, lodging, meals, and treatment for about $1,414 during the summer season (take-home material is not included). Interested? Write Romanian National Tourist Office, 573 Third Avenue, New York, New York 10016.

Meanwhile, I've been hearing reports of great strides being made in rejuvenation by a Finnish scientist working on a large grant from a giant American pharmaceutical company, so whether you call it *rejuvenation* or *revitalization,* this is big business.

FACIAL ISOMETRICS

Will facial exercises help stave off wrinkles and firm up facial contours? The American Medical Association says no, contending that no facial exercise, isometric or otherwise, will help because while facial muscles can be exercised, the aging is due mostly to the skin's losing its elasticity.

Still, there are plenty of men who do facial isometrics faithfully every day, take note of the temporary glow it gives their skin, and feel and look refreshed. If they haven't stretched the skin in the process, I see no reason why they shouldn't continue doing them. The problem is that unless done properly, the twitching, winking, mugging motions can create lines.

Now I won't say that the following set of facial exercises will retard the aging process, but I do know that they stimulate the circulation and appear to plump up the skin so that for a short time afterward your face does look better. Try these exercises, but before you do, I suggest you apply a moisturizer to the skin of your face and neck and open your shirt collar and loosen your tie. And do them before a mirror so that you're absolutely certain your control fingers are properly placed.

For the Chin

You remember those caricatures of Maurice Chevalier emphasizing the protruding lower lip? That's the general idea here. Lift your chin, and imagine you're trying to touch the tip of your nose with your lower lip. You'll feel the pull in both chin and neck muscles. Do at least ten repetitions.

Place the length of your tongue against the roof of your mouth, and press. This gives a lift to the underchin. Do it ten times.

For the Neck

One sure sign of aging is the cord or "canal" that starts showing up in the center of the neck. Here's an antidote for it: Stick your tongue out as far as it will go, and then aim up toward the tip of your nose. Do six times.

Try to grin without parting your lips. Your mouth will try to curve up at the corners, but resist the movement. That way your neck muscles will flex from your earlobes clear down to the base of your throat. Do ten times.

For the Mouth

As we age, our lips often lose their shape and vertical lines etch their way into the skin above the upper lip. The following exercise is designed to discourage all that.

Say the word "church" in a slow, exaggerated way. This will lift your lips up and forward until the two tips of your upper lip peak. Do this exercise ten times.

For the Jawline

Place three fingers of your right hand on the left side of your face so that they extend from the corner of the left nostril down to the corner of your mouth (the nasal-labial fold). Now gently press your left thumb on the outside of your left eye and the remaining fingers of your left hand on the area just above and between your eyebrows; these are the control fingers strategically placed to prevent lines from forming as you do this face-lift exercise.

With control fingers in place but not pressing down on the skin, wink your left eye as you lift the left side of your mouth. It's a wink-and-grin combination that should be executed *fast*. Do fifty times, taking care to wink and grin simultaneously.

Repeat fifty times on the right side of your face by reversing your hands.

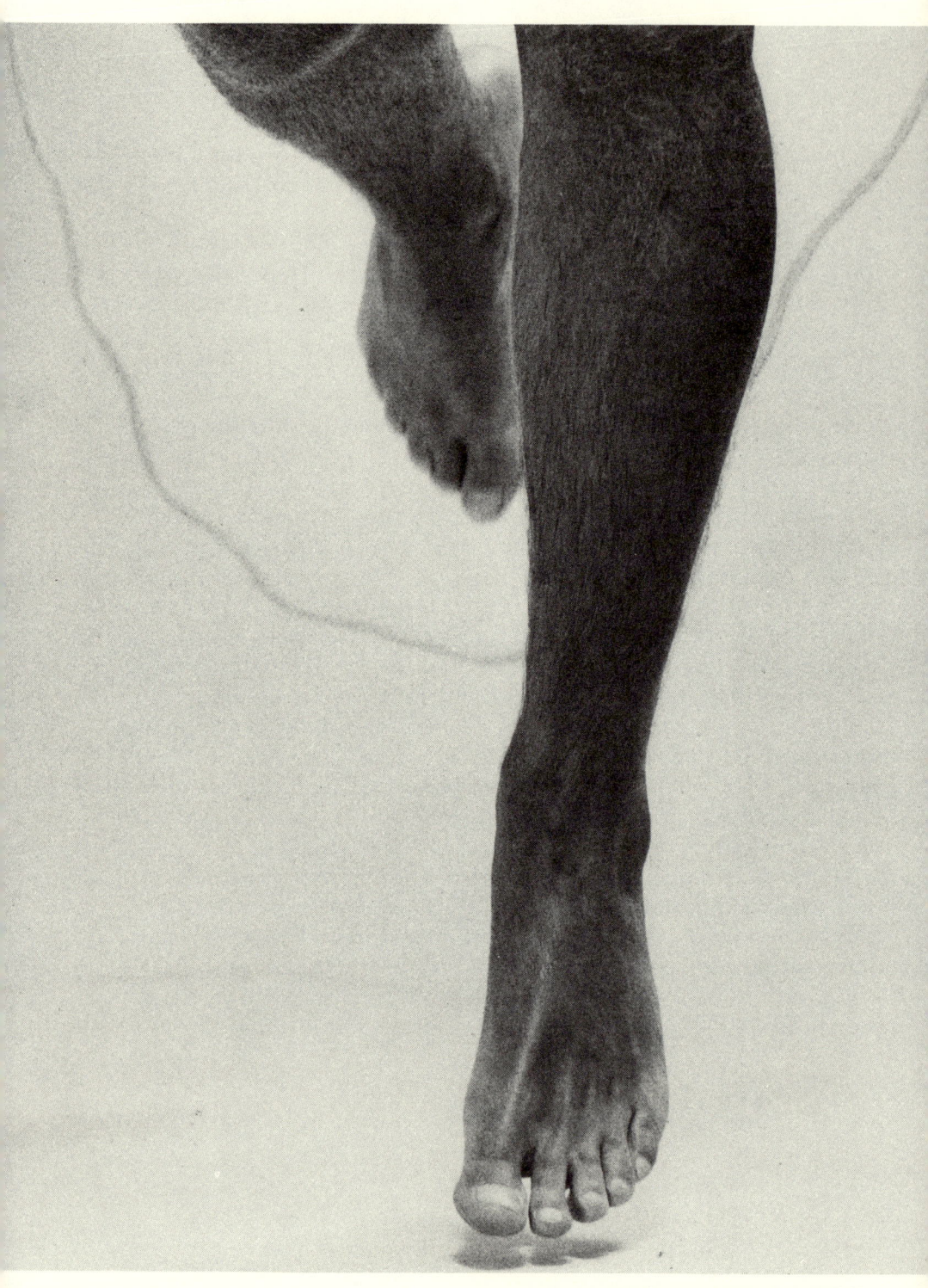

PHOTO BY ROBERT EPSTEIN.

For Strong, Nimble Legs and Feet

FOOTNOTES

One-fourth of all the bones in your body are in your feet, 26 in all, intricately linked by 33 joints and tied together with 200 ligaments. It's small wonder that feet are considered a masterpiece of structural engineering.

The average man walks 165,000 miles during his lifetime, and his feet absorb a cumulative total pressure of some 1,000 tons a day. Under the circumstances, it's amazing to me that we tend to take our pedal extremities so for granted. Women pay more attention to their feet, possibly because they have more foot problems since they spend most of their waking hours tottering around on high heels. A man's feet have an easier time of it. They're encased in more sensible shoes, and he walks in closer contact with the ground, all of which must be rather reassuring to a pair of appendages situated at the southern tip of the anatomy. Yet in World War II three-fourths of inductees examined for fitness had something wrong with their feet. So while men don't squeeze theirs into high-heeled shoes, we often adopt a cavalier attitude when it comes to fit. Year after year we buy the same size, not bothering to have our feet measured, and while it's true that feet stop growing around age eighteen, a change in weight or change in exercise patterns can change foot measurements. Actually foot measurements change in the course of the day every day, a fact which leads Dr. Rob Roy McGregor, a podiatrist and medical adviser to the Footwear Council, to advise that you shop for shoes around midday, when you've been on your feet a few hours and they're at their fullest. Sometimes the difference can be as much as one whole size.

Still, it's not your shoes but how you walk—briskly, erectly, confidently—that indicates your youthfulness. And that's possible only with healthy, well-cared-for feet.

FOOT CARE

It's never too late to start, and to quote famed nutritionist-writer Gayelord Hauser, more agile at eighty-four than most men half his age, "It will pay better dividends in youthfulness than a facial massage, a fancy necktie, or an afternoon at the races."

It's not for nothing that it's said we wear our shoes on our faces. Imprison your feet in a pair of ill-fitting shoes, and you wear their pain on your face. Remember, you should be able to wiggle your toes in any pair of shoes you buy; that means there should be an absolute minimum of a quarter of an inch between the front of the shoe and your longest toe.

At least one night a week treat your feet like the good sports they are. Line up the following allies: a foot soap, a camphored cream for massaging, a cooling talcum powder, a toenail clipper and file, and a pumice stone—and go to it!

1. Fill a basin with hot water, into which you pour Johnson's foot soap (despite the name, it's actually a powder that dissolves instantly upon contact with the water). Relax, and soak for fifteen to twenty minutes.

2. Using the pumice stone, smooth the skin on the backs of your heels and the bottoms of your feet, which on many a man's foot is layered with a hide that would do an elephant proud.

3. Towel dry, and with your toenail clipper, cut your nails straight across, slightly below the tip of the toe. If you cut away the sides of the nails, you're encouraging ingrown toenails.

4. File nails smooth.

5. Now comes the most satisfying part of all. Massage with the camphored cream. Don't rush. Start by kneading the sole with your fist; move on to a fingertip rubbing of the ankle and heel, squeeze the entire foot between your hands, and finish with a twisting massage of each toe.

6. Sprinkle on some cooling talc between the toes and on the soles of your feet. One podiatrist I know recommends daily use of talcum powder, considering it the most important bit of advice he can give a patient since feet are almost always a trifle damp, and trapped between toes, this dampness can lead to fungal and bacterial infections.

SORE FEET

It's estimated that seven out of ten adult Americans have sore feet. Bone surgery is required for some of the more serious foot problems, but usually a visit to a podiatrist will solve most sore foot problems

Blisters, for example, are caused by constant friction—caused mostly by ill-fitting shoes. Often you can treat a blister yourself by soaking your foot in a pint of warm water to which you've added a teaspoon of table salt. Do that for ten to fifteen minutes a couple of times a day, and the blister will very likely disappear.

Corns and calluses are also the result of abnormal pressure and friction. Assuming that your foot is otherwise normal and a shoe is the culprit, you might buy one of the over-the-counter products designed to soften corns and calluses. Since skin is constantly being shed, a softened callus will usually fall off, but a corn has a hard core, and consequently, it's more difficult to treat. If you can't get to a podiatrist right away, you can alleviate some of the discomfort by the use of either a doughnut-shaped piece of felt or a piece of foam rubber, the idea being to prevent any further rubbing of skin against shoe. I don't recommend your investing in any of the over-the-counter corn removers.

The bony bump known as a bunion sometimes is caused by ill-fitting shoes and sometimes is a matter of heredity. Faulty foot construction can cause the bones and muscles in the feet to carry more than their rightful share of body weight, and as a result, a bunion grows. Now, however, there's an operation that solves the problem in under forty-five minutes. Novocaine is administered via compressed air, and a high-speed dentist's drill powers a bone-cutting bur that removes the dastardly bunion (without stitches), after which the foot is bandaged up to the ankle and the patient is able to walk out of the doctor's office. The approximate cost is $500 per foot, and this includes postsurgical care.

VARICOSE VEINS

They certainly don't help a man cut a dashing figure at the beach or poolside. Varicose veins are caused by a variety of things, and the warning signs are several:

Inflammation of veins in the legs
Feeling of heaviness in the legs
Dull stabbing pain in the legs
Leg cramps at night
Itching around the ankles
Tenderness and soreness along the veins

Treatment varies from wearing tailor-made elastic hose to injections. In severe cases, a physician may recommend surgery.

What Can You Do to Avoid Varicose Veins?

... When sitting, elevate your legs.

... On long trips don't forget to get up and stretch your legs.

... Never wear round garters for long periods of time.

... Stimulate circulation by exercising. Sluggish circulation in the legs is a contributing cause of varicose veins. Walking is the best and simplest exercise since it causes leg muscles to contract.

Great circulation boosters, too, are foot-and-leg exercises, and here are some that I guarantee will help put spring in your step. Do them without shoes and socks.

1. *For ankles.* Sit straight on a straight-back chair with a leg crossed over the knee of the opposite leg. Bend the crossed leg down, in toward the ankle, and then up. Do ten times and then another ten times, but now reversing the direction of the circle. Repeat this exercise with the other leg.

2. *For arches.* Stand with both feet pointing straight ahead, from six to eight inches apart. Rise on your toes, and slowly, to the count of ten, return to the starting position. Do ten repetitions.

3. *For ankles and arches.* Rise on your toes, just as you did in the previous exercise, but now roll your feet outward and back onto the heel twenty times so that your full weight comes on the outside of your feet and both the inner and under parts of your feet lift clear off the floor. Do six repetitions.

4. *For arch and leg muscles.* Sit on the floor with your legs straight ahead, and without bending your knees, turn the soles of your feet closely together. Do ten repetitions.

5. *For calves.* Stand about three feet from a wall, and place both palms flat against the wall. Turn toes inward, and roll the weight of your body to the outside edges of your feet. Do ten repetitions.

6. *For toes and feet.* Stand with feet parallel, and curl toes up-

ward as far as possible and then return to the floor slowly. Do ten repetitions.

COMMENTARY

A lot of what passes for foot care is just plain common sense.

. . . Give your feet sun, air, and freedom from constriction. Walk barefoot whenever possible on a slightly yielding surface, like sand or grass.

. . . Wear clean socks, and slip a pair of odor-destroying insoles into your shoes (Johnson's Odor-Eaters, for instance) that will absorb perspiration.

. . . When walking, place your whole foot on the ground, first heel, then toes—with toes pointed neither in nor out but straight ahead. Never walk on your toes; this puts a strain on calves and ankles.

. . . Wear the shoes that were specially designed for your particular sport. Don't wear your tennis shoes for jogging and vice versa.

. . . And when nobody's around, swing both feet up onto the top of your desk and relax!

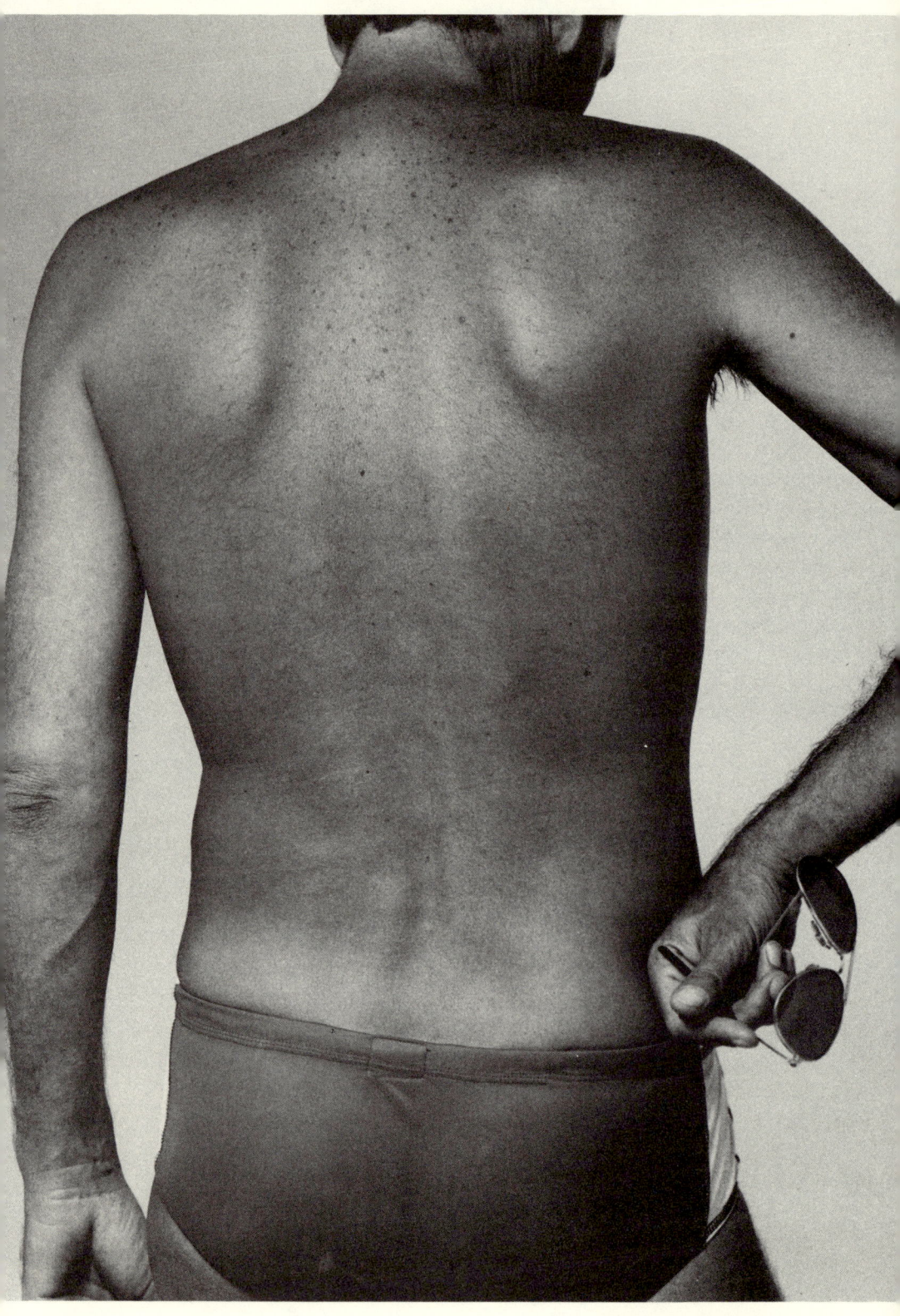

PHOTO BY ROBERT EPSTEIN.

For a Straight, Pain-Free Back and Firm, Flat Stomach

"People really don't stoop because they're old," says C. Carson Conrad, executive director of the President's Council on Physical Fitness and Sports. "They're old because they stoop." One of the chief reasons they do is an aching back, and they don't have to be over forty to suffer from one. Backaches today are so commonplace that they've assumed epidemic proportions; that is why in 1976 the YMCA established "The Y's Way to a Healthy Back" as a national program.

Of course, there are many causes of backaches—underexercise and overstress, for instance. Some backaches are easily remedied—some by simply improving posture. Others require medical attention because the backache is merely a symptom of underlying disease. The most common cause of backache in older men comes about simply through the wear and tear of aging. "But you can't give in to it—you just have to work your way through it and stretch and stretch," advises Conrad. Stretching relaxes the muscles and pulls the spine, thus making a man able to maintain a more upright posture and have better muscular strength to maintain the skeletal structure. Dr. Willibald Nagler, physiatrist-in-chief at the New York Hospital–Cornell Medical Center, says there's an old Hungarian adage that applies: "Young people are made by God. Older people make themselves." In short, *you* program the way your body looks; by the way you stand, sit, and walk, you become the sculptor of your own body.

How can you help prevent your backaches? The following lifestyle habits will go a long way toward preventing lower backache and other back pains:

1. Exercise regularly to keep your muscles strong—especially the abdominal muscles so important to back support.

2. Stand tall, with your chin and abdomen tucked in, your back as straight as possible.

3. When standing in one place for a lengthy period of time, put one foot up on the rung of a chair, box, or other object.

4. Your mattress should be firm but flexible enough that it adjusts to the natural contours of your body.

5. When driving, have the seat forward enough to keep your knees bent and lower back straight. (When a car seat's too far back, legs are almost straight and the lower back is curved.)

6. Sit well back in chairs, with your back straight. Don't slouch.

7. Try to sleep on your side, with knees bent, or on your back with a pillow under your knees. *Don't* sleep on your stomach.

8. Don't stay in one position all day, such as at a desk. Get up now and then to stretch and walk about.

9. Lift things by stooping—that is, bend your knees and keep your back straight.

10. Hold objects that you're carrying as close to your body as possible.

So far as I'm concerned, Rule Number 2 can't be stressed too much. Proper posture not only can prevent or alleviate backache but does wonders for appearance as well. I've seen many a man look slimmer when in reality he actually hadn't lost a pound; he had lost inches because proper posture had put his body in alignment—

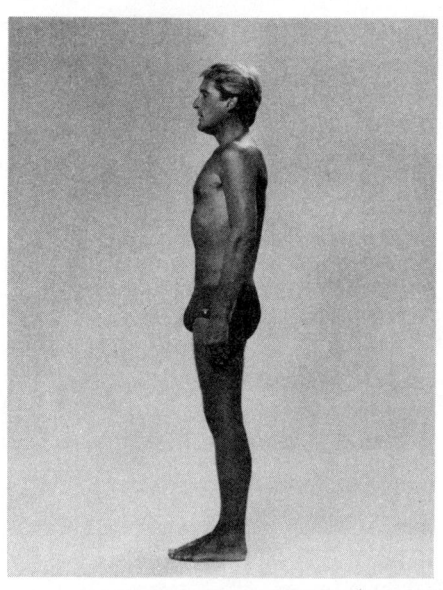

PHOTO BY ROBERT EPSTEIN.

hips swung under the spine, knees and ankles directly in line with the hips. Presto! His waistline was stretched, and his stomach flattened, and an incipient second chin disappeared in the process. Good posture can trim the body; poor posture can give even a thin man a potbelly. No amount of dieting or exercise is going to correct our body faults if we're not stacked in proper alignment.

Always be aware of your posture—standing, sitting, walking. Good posture can't be a sometime thing. Make a conscious effort at first, and prety soon good posture habits will come automatically. Then you'll feel lighter and more energetic, while you also help keep your back from getting out of whack.

Now here's the simplest way I know to put your body in balance:

> Stand with your back, head, and shoulders against a wall, heels about one inch away from the wall and toes pointing straight ahead. At that point you're in perfect alignment, so close your eyes, and concentrate on how it feels. Then walk away from the wall, imagining that it is still behind you.

Until perfect posture comes naturally to you, during the course of the day check up on yourself; take inventory of your body parts. Once you understand how one part relates to another (rather like lifting the hood of a car and having a look at the mechanics of what makes it go), you'll be better able to appreciate what good body mechanics are all about. The following body-inventory exercise will do that for you, unobtrusively, in something like eight seconds flat.

> Stand with feet a few inches apart, toes pointing straight ahead. Slowly draw the buttocks tightly together. Then distribute your weight evenly on both legs by pressing on the ball of each foot. Tighten the muscles in front of your thighs. Then slowly stretch the spine; imagine that you're trying to touch the ceiling with the crown of your head, but don't tilt your chin in the process. Don't raise your shoulders, but draw your shoulder blades together, and allow both arms to hang loosely at your sides.

Good posture isn't sucking in your breath, pulling your shoulders up, and sticking your chin out, nor is it a stiff-armed, stiff-backed military stance. Good posture is simply putting the parts of your body in balance, one to the other, so that you use *all* your muscles in the way they were intended to be used according to the laws of body mechanics. That way no one part of your body—your back, for example—is forced to do more than its rightful share of the work.

Dr. Nagler maintains that strong abdominal muscles are essential if a man is to have a strong, pain-free back. The following ten exercises,* many of which involve s-t-r-e-t-c-h-i-n-g, have been designed to strengthen the back or abdomen and, in some instances, both at the same time. Note that most of the exercises done while you lie on your back on the floor require that your knees be bent and that way take any possible strain off the back muscles. In fact, the best way I know to rest your back is to lie on the floor in this position.

1. Lie on your back with knees bent, feet flat on the floor, and arms at your sides. Push the small of your back into the floor by pinching your buttocks together and pulling in your stomach until it's flat against the floor. Breathe out as you do this by counting out loud to six. Let go. Repeat six times.

2. Lie on your back with knees bent, feet flat on the floor, and arms at your sides. Begin to exhale slowly while you lift your head only far enough so that you can see your navel. Exhale by counting out loud to six. Return to starting position, gently rolling your head from side to side. Repeat six times.

3. Lying on your back with knees bent, feet flat on the floor, bring both knees up to your chest. Hug each leg below the knee, and slowly pull both knees up as close as you can to your chest. Count to six, and return legs to starting position. Do six repetitions.

4. Lie on your back, this time with knees bent and arms straight at your sides, palms down. Lift your chest until your back is off the floor. The important thing here is not to give yourself any assist with your hands. Slowly return to starting position. Repeat five times.

5. Lie flat on the floor with both arms straight at your sides, palms down. Keeping knees stiff, lift both legs up and over your head, and attempt to touch the floor while keeping arms and back flat on the floor. Hold this position to the count of five. Relax, and return to starting position. Repeat five times.

6. Lie on your back with hands behind your neck and legs bent, feet flat on the floor. Slowly rise up off the floor, while at the same time bending your head and neck and curving your back. Continue until your forehead touches your knees. Hold this position to the

---

*Numbers 1, 2, 7, and 9 were developed by the Department of Rehabilitation Medicine at the New York Hospital–Cornell Medical Center.

count of five, and then slowly return to starting position. Do ten repetitions.

7. Kneel on the floor with both hands underneath your shoulders, palms down on the floor. Knees should be shoulder width apart and elbows straight throughout the entire exercise. Drop your head, pull in your stomach muscles, and try to get your back as round and high as possible. Exhale while assuming this position to the count of five. Inhale as you raise your head up and return to starting position. Do five repetitions.

8. Start in the kneeling position, drop your head forward, bend both elbows, and extend your arms forward until they are straight out and your forehead touches the floor. As you do this, arch your back so that your buttocks are as high as you can get them. Hold this position to the count of five. Relax, and return to starting position. Do five repetitions.

9. Standing with feet about six inches apart, bend knees slightly; reach down, and rest your hands on your thighs. Pull in your stomach while counting out loud to five. Let go. Repeat five times.

10. Stand facing a wall with feet together and toes about three feet from the base of the wall. Now lean forward so that the palms of both hands are flat against the wall; your hands should be level with your shoulders and a shoulder width apart. With both feet flat on the floor, allow yourself to sink toward the wall while keeping your back straight; your elbows will protrude to the side. Push away from the wall, and let your back sway, still keeping both palms flat against the wall. Drop your head down as far as you can without changing the position of your hands and feet. Lead with your chin, and raise your head up; as you do this, your back will arch. Do this exercise five times.

Remember: Poor posture puts a strain on the lower back; overweight puts a strain on the lower back; back problems can respond to exercise.

Dr. Hans Kraus, an orthopedic physician who developed the YMCA's "Healthy Back" program, shows a color slide of a friend of his who, at seventy-one, is still climbing mountains. Exercise helped him heal and got him back into shape after a sixty-foot fall.

If your backaches persist, see your doctor.

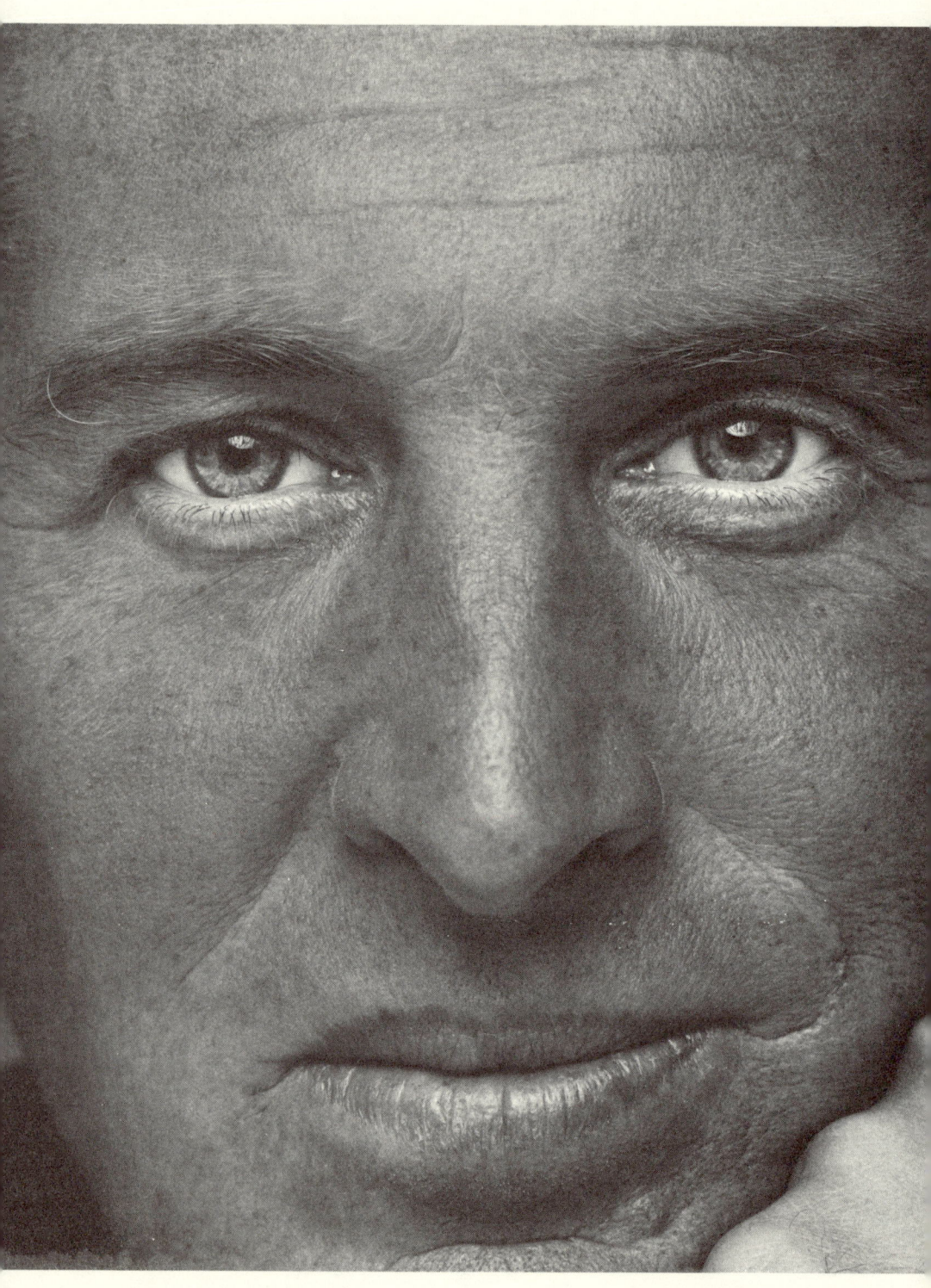

PHOTO BY ROBERT EPSTEIN.

For Clear, Youthful-Looking Eyes

Without a doubt, your eyes are the hardest-working part of you. Except when you're sleeping, your eyes are working, and 365 days of hard work plus pollution, bouts of too little sleep, and often a nutritionally poor diet can take their toll.

According to Dr. Morgan B. Raiford, medical director of the Atlanta Eye Clinic, eyes are affected first and most dramatically by a nutritionally poor diet. Forty-five percent of Americans are said to have some form of visual defect, a great proportion of which are nutrition-related. To keep eyes healthy and vision good, a person needs a diet containing 25 to 30 percent whole protein, which is about three times as much meat, fish, and eggs as he now consumes: Says Dr. Raiford, "only about ten percent of the average American's daily intake of food is protein, and the balance is worthless starchy and sugary food items." As a result, "the blood vessels leading to the retina in the eye get all clogged up by those sugars, fats, and starches and can't supply the photoelectric cells of the retina. The retina eventually becomes starved from lack of fuel."

CATARACTS

A gradual loss of clearness, or transparency, of the lens of the eye, the cataract is the most important single cause of blindness among adults today. With aging, the lens in almost everybody's eyes becomes slightly hazy, but when it becomes cloudy, a cataract is developing, and this can lead to blindness if not treated. Furthermore, if you develop a cataract in one eye, you are very likely to develop one in your other eye later.

What can be done? A cataract can be detected by an ophthalmologist during a regular eye examination—one more reason why a man over forty should have his eyes examined once every year. Once a cataract develops, the only satisfactory treatment is the removal of the cloudy lens by surgery. There are no eye drops, salves, or medicines to treat cataracts. It's heartening to note that 95 percent of cataract surgery is successful and the patient's vision is restored.

GLAUCOMA

This is the second leading cause of blindness in America, and it afflicts more than 1 million Americans over the age of thirty-five. Glaucoma is caused by an increase in pressure inside the eye, and in time this abnormally high eye pressure will permanently destroy the nerve cells. A person may have glaucoma for months or years before experiencing any difficulties. Mysteriously it usually strikes people whose eyes are healthy. Although the cause of glaucoma is unknown, it can be controlled if found early and treated properly. Each year have your eye doctor check you for it.

GLASSES versus CONTACT LENSES

Farsightedness seems to come with age, and as a result, most men forty and over wear glasses at least some of the time or, I should say, wear glasses or contact lenses. The choice is usually cosmetic, although not everyone should or can wear contacts. But most eye doctors believe that contact lenses actually improve vision more than glasses do.

What about hard contact lenses versus the new soft ones? The soft are almost always more comfortable, but the hard ones are said generally to give better vision. Soft lenses won't pop out or trap foreign particles since they're fitted intimately to the eye, and since they don't alter the shape of the cornea, there's no blur if you change from lenses to glasses. But the soft contacts do demand a little more in the way of maintenance (being boiled every night in their special apparatus, for example), and they do damage more easily than hard contacts.

So far as glasses go, yours should do more than improve your vision; they should also improve your looks. And they will if you choose the proper frames for your shape face.

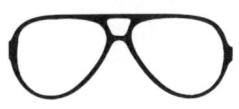 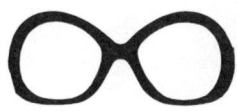 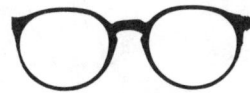

For a Square Face

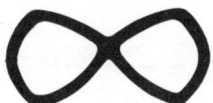 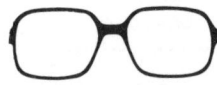 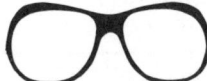

For a Long Face

 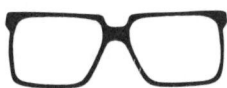 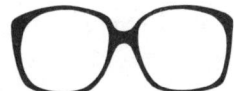

For a Round Face

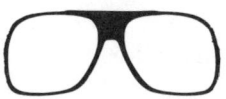  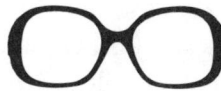

For an Oval Face

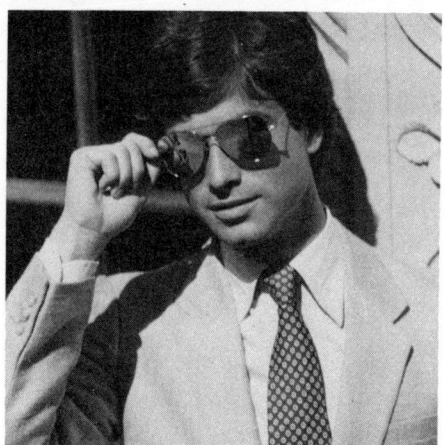

PHOTO COURTESY OF FOSTER GRANT.

SUNGLASSES

The right frame, the right tint, the right style—and then you've got a pair, sleek and functional, that will give you high-level protection from glare, wind, dust, and soot.

Actually the bigger the frames, the better. The frames and lenses should cover your whole field of vision, and your glasses should be dark enough to cut brightness, but not too dark—that puts another kind of strain on the eyes.

Plastic versus glass? That's strictly a matter of personal preference. True, plastic scratches more easily than glass, but if you choose glass, be sure it's *safety* glass, which crumbles rather than shatters if it breaks. Government regulations now call for shatter-resistant glass; check for the sticker.

The most recommended sunglass colors are gray, smoke, green-gray, and brown, and the more neutral the lens color, the less distortion of colors around you.

When you select your sunglasses, here's a quick test for quality: Stand under a fluorescent fixture, hold the glasses with the light reflecting on the inside lens, and move slightly. If image is distorted, the lenses are faulty and will cause strain.

RED EYE

Natural tearing of the eyes is the best eyewash. Next best are eyedrops and eyewashes. Some doctors are leery of eyedrops' being used too often, the thought being that you may become addicted to them and find yourself forced to use more and more to get rid of the red. But when I queried an eye specialist about that, his reply was: "No one's ever OD'd on eyedrops!" Still, he did allow that an eyewash is perhaps preferable to drops and has a brief soothing effect as well.

A proven way to relax tired eyes is to take a couple of sterile gauze pads or cotton balls, dampen them with witch hazel, place them on your closed eyes, and stretch out for about fifteen minutes.

When you've had too much of close paperwork, turn around and stare out the window at the farthest object you can see; that's eyeball-stretching. When you've had enough of that, cup a hand over each eye so that no light can enter, and sit and stare into the blackness for a couple of minutes—very, very refreshing.

DYEING LASHES AND BROWS

Most men will adjust more readily to gray hair than they will to gray lashes and brows. Good reason, too, for once the small hairs framing the eyes lose their color, the eyes look washed out, lose their prominence. Dyeing them every four to six weeks is usually enough to keep youthful color in and gray out.

The whole procedure, brows and lashes, takes about one hour. The dye is applied with a special orange stick or Q-Tip first to the bottom lashes of both eyes and then to the upper lashes. While they're drying, the colorist applies a lighter shade of dye to the brows for a more natural look. The dye, which contains only about 1 percent peroxide, won't smudge or wash off.

THE EYE-LIFT

Taking out bags under eyes or excising the crepey or drooping eyelid has become commonplace. Sometimes it's done as part of a complete face-lift, but done by itself, it's minor surgery, and recovery time is the fastest of any form of cosmetic surgery. And since the upper half of the face stretches and sags less than the lower half of the face, results are longer-lasting.

The fine sutures come out in two to four days, sometimes earlier. Healing time is about ten days, but with sunglasses concealing his swollen eyes, a man can resume normal activities almost immediately. Ordinarily an eye-lift lasts five to seven years, and smoothing out bags under the eyes is usually a permanent improvement.

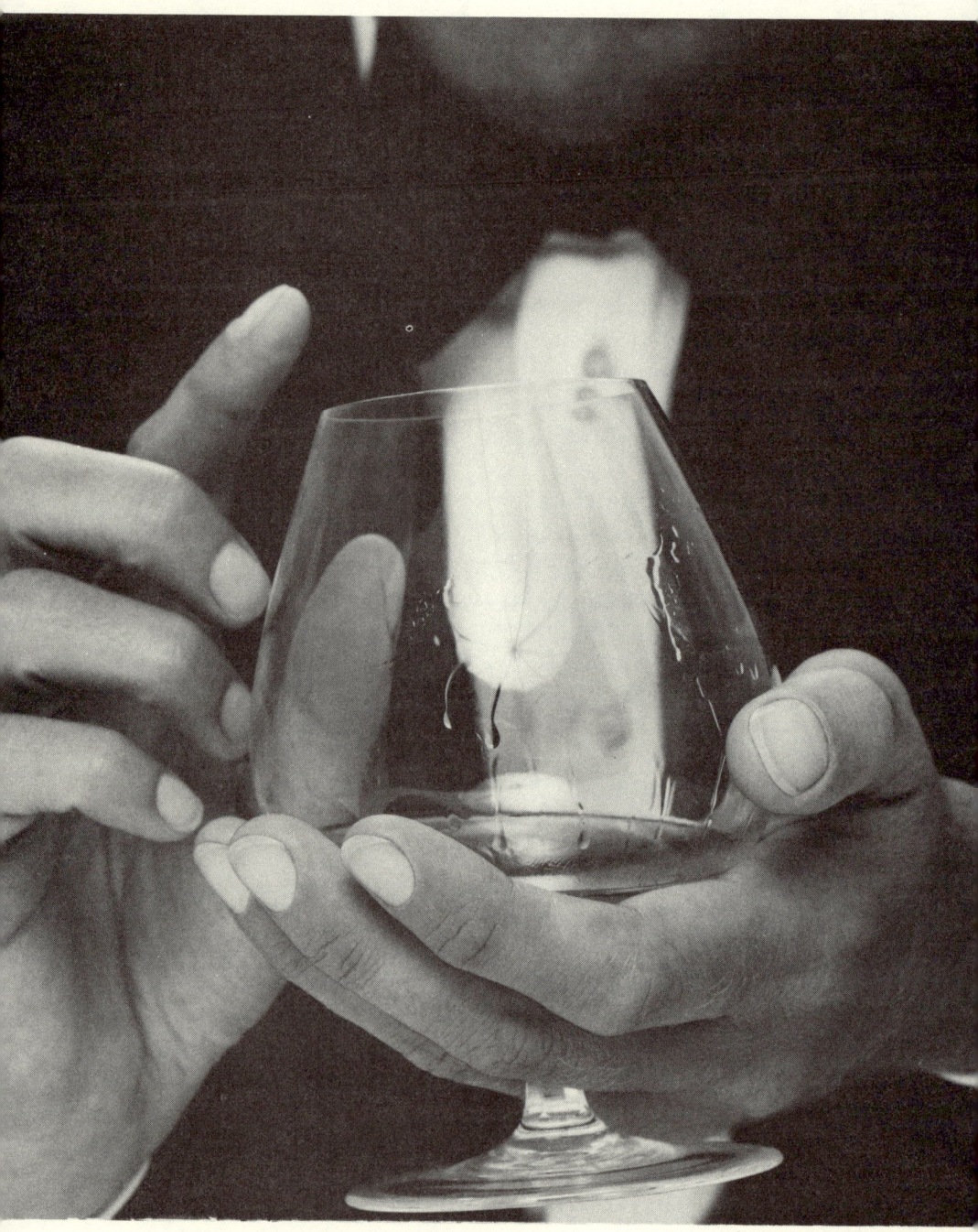

PHOTO BY ROBERT EPSTEIN.

For Smooth Hands and Strong Nails

Your head and hands are on permanent display. Yet many a man who's into skin care for his face doesn't do anything for his hands except wash them. And there's the rub! The skin on your hands has fewer oil cells than that on your face, and since in the course of a day a man washes his hands more often than his face, the tops of the hands become dry and sometimes rough and red. When that happens, apply a hand cream or lotion—at least before bedtime—and during cold weather, protect your hands and prevent chapping by wearing gloves; in the winter gloves are more than a fashion accessory—they're a necessity.

Hand care can be pleasantly minimal because hands respond quickly to good treatment, and well-cared-for hands say nice things about a man—that he cares about himself right down to his fingertips, for example.

A professional manicure now and then will do as much for your self-esteem as it will for your nails. But you can give yourself a dandy manicure at home and save the $5 or $6 plus tip. It's simple. Start by laying out a hand towel, on which you line up the following: a small dish filled with warm, soapy water, an emery board, a nailbrush, an orangewood stick, cotton balls, petroleum jelly, hand cream or lotion, cuticle scissors, and a chamois buffer.

1. Start by filing your nails with the smooth side of the emery board; it's easier on nails than a metal file. Don't saw back and forth, but file in one direction, gently. Avoid filing deeply into the corners because this weakens nails; in fact, simply round off the tops of your nails, and don't touch the sides. The secret of strong nails is to let them grow straight at the sides. (Nails grow 70 percent faster on fingers than on toes.)

2. Next, soak your nails in the warm, soapy water, and with your nailbrush remove cuticles from the surface of the nails. Wipe dry, and with the hand towel gently push the cuticles back.

3. You want the moon of each nail to show clear and white, so rub each cuticle with some of the petroleum jelly, and then, with

the moistened orangewood stick wrapped in cotton, gently lift and push it back.

4. Now, with the cotton-tipped orangewood stick, clean under each nail, and then wipe nails clean with a cotton ball to remove all traces of oil.

5. Massage your hand cream or lotion into both wrists and hands, using a kneading motion.

6. Hangnails? Remove them with your cuticle scissors.

7. Whether or not you use a clear, colorless nail polish is up to you. If you do, start at the base of the nail and use firm upward strokes. Three strokes are recommended: one from the base to the tip at the center of the nail and then one stroke on each side of the nail. There should be enough polish on the brush to complete one nail without redipping. Take care not to touch the cuticle with the polish.

8. Polish or no polish, finish with a chamois buffer to give your nails a handsome, low-key shine.

NAIL STRENGTHENERS

Knox gelatin is said to be one. Add water to the contents of a packet, stir, and swallow—and your nails will grow strong. At least that's what I hear, but I'm not convinced. Gelatin is said to provide protein, but it's not a complete one; it actually provides barely more than 50 percent. Better to get your high-quality protein and calcium in your diet than to rely on a packet of gelatin.

For a nail strengthener, I prefer to mix a little white iodine and olive oil and with a Q-Tip apply it directly to the entire nail, leaving a thin film on overnight.

AGE SPOTS

Age spots are also known as liver spots, although there's absolutely no connection between them and liver disease. They're also occasionally called senile freckles, although there's no connection whatsoever with senility. Those frecklelike brown spots come with age all right, but usually after years of unwise exposure to sun and wind. Can you rid your hands of them? Yes and no. While you can't actually make them totally disappear, you can use a hand cream containing hydroquinone to lighten them significantly. Since this chemical causes allergic reactions in some individuals, it's recommended that you take a patch test before using a cream with it.

FIVE-FINGER EXERCISE

It's not only the skin on hands that shows age. Stiff fingers do, too. The best way I know to keep your fingers flexible is exercise.

1. Make a fist, hold it tightly, and then fling your hand open with all fingers spread.
2. Take a rubber ball, and squeeze it as though you were trying to puncture it with your fingers.
3. Open your hand wide, and starting with your index finger, bring each finger firmly into contact with your thumb.

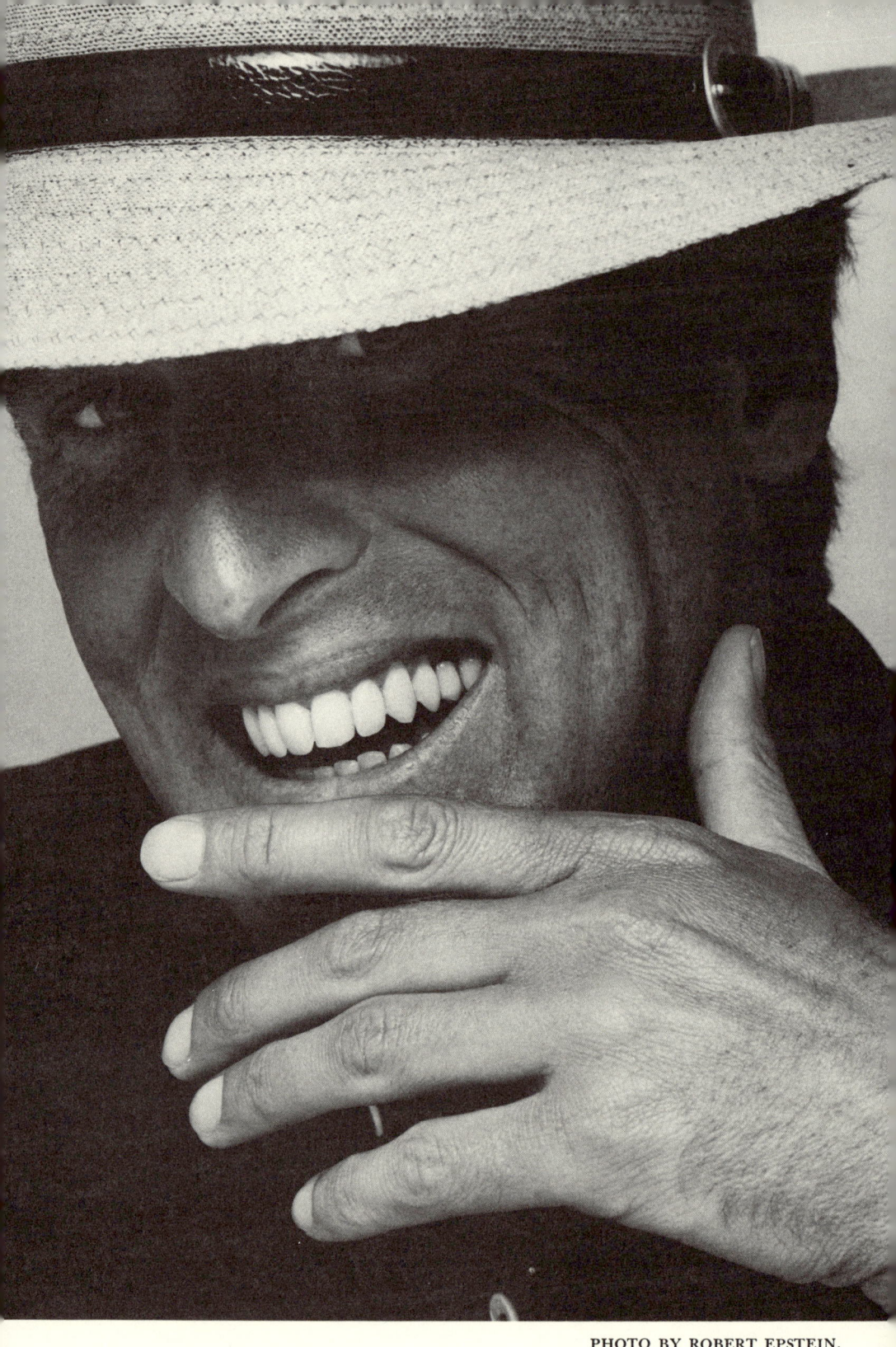

PHOTO BY ROBERT EPSTEIN.

For a Winning Smile

You've heard the expression "long in the tooth"? It means *old*. But do you know its origin? Not surprisingly it's rooted in the mouth. As the gum recedes from the neck of a tooth, the jawbone—where teeth are supported—is also affected and joins in the retreat, leaving more and more of the tooth exposed, hence a longer-looking tooth.

A man doesn't have to be, say, past forty in order to qualify as "long in the tooth." Twenty million Americans suffer from such periodontal ("around the tooth") disease, and most of them have had the beginnings of it by the age of fifteen. Nearly 23 million people in this country have lost all their teeth despite the fact that tooth enamel is the hardest substance in the human body.

The cure? *Preventive dentistry.* While periodontal (gum) disease, the most common cause of tooth loss, is insidious (it's nearly always painless in its early stages), it's also almost entirely avoidable if you practice preventive dentistry.

  . . . Eat less sugar.
  . . . Brush and floss properly.
  . . . See your dentist every six months.

Bacteria in the mouth thrive on sugar-rich foods, converting the residue—a scant fifteen minutes after you've taken your first bite—to produce a substance called dextran that helps bacteria cling to teeth. Result: *plaque*, a gummy, colorless film which, unless it's removed every twenty-four to thirty-six hours, can harden into calculus—hard tartar—which leads to swollen, inflamed gums that recede from the teeth, allowing the bacteria to move down along the roots of the teeth to the bone sockets. The rest of the story you already know: The teeth loosen and fall out. So the plot goes like this: Sugar plus Bacteria plus Plaque equals not only holes in the teeth but, all too often, holes in the gums the teeth once occupied. (It's also interesting to note that there's a high incidence of cavities among men who have quit smoking; it seems that many of them switch to chewing gum and candy to take the place of the missing weed.)

A few years ago medical researchers at Cornell University reported that many patients with periodontal disease have shown evidence of osteoporosis, a malady that makes bones porous and brittle as we grow older. When it attacks the mouth, it means destruction of the bony supports of the teeth. An insufficient intake of calcium is a major contributing cause. Your bones and teeth are constructed mostly of calcium, and the U.S. Public Health Service recommends that anyone over forty get a high calcium supply in his diet to promote bone strength. A very important part of your preventive dentistry program should be to increase your calcium intake by drinking skim milk every day; milk and milk products are a primary source of calcium. If you dislike drinking milk, you may want to consider bone meal as a dietary supplement; it is simply the powdered bones of young beef cattle, nothing more, nothing less, and is available in tablet form.

CLEANING YOUR TEETH

When I was a boy, the accepted technique for cleaning teeth was use of a vigorous back-and-forth motion with the toothbrush, taking care not to brush the gums. The most you could do to the gums was massage them with the pad of your forefinger; anything else was said to irritate them. Well, everything changes with time—even the way you brush your teeth and exercise your gums.

Today cleaning your teeth is a two-part program: dental floss to clean between the teeth where a brush can't reach and a special brushing technique, using an up-and-down motion. Some men brush first and then floss, but I recommend the reverse, thereby letting the brush sweep away what the flossing dislodges. It's best, of course, to brush after every meal and every between-meal snack, but it's absolutely essential that you floss and brush thoroughly at least once a day for plaque not to harden.

Choose the *unwaxed* dental floss. It's more abrasive and this is essential for cleaning between teeth. Snap off an eighteen-inch piece, and wrap the ends around the middle fingers of each hand, holding a section of about one and a half inches between the thumbs and forefingers. Holding the floss tightly—in other words, no slack—gently, with a kind of sawing motion, ease it down through the tight place between the teeth. *Don't* snap it down, or you're apt to cut into the gum. Once the floss reaches the gumline, curve it into a C shape around the tooth, slide it into the space between the gum and the tooth, and move it up and down against the side of the tooth. That done, curve it around the neighboring tooth, and repeat. Ease the floss back out through the teeth, and repeat on the next pair of teeth, using a clean section of floss. Continue this way until all your teeth, top and bottom, have been flossed. Then rinse your mouth to wash out the bacteria you've loosened, and you're ready to brush.

Choose a soft brush with rounded-end bristles and a flat brushing surface. An electric toothbrush? Dandy, although most dentists I've talked to prefer the old-fashioned toothbrush for more versatility of action and better cleaning. But remember, a worn-out toothbrush can't effectively clean your teeth, so trade in one with loose or bent bristles for a new model.

Steer clear of highly abrasive toothpastes and powders. Tooth powders are the most abrasive. Anyway, no paste or powder can whiten teeth since it doesn't contain a bleach. What it can do, however, is polish and brighten teeth, and that's no little improvement.

Fluoride is a chemical compound that makes teeth more resistant to decay, and despite the fact that cavities are less common after the age of twenty-five, I recommend a fluoride toothpaste, unless you're one of the 100 million Americans who enjoy the benefits of fluoridated water. Look for a toothpaste carrying the seal of the American Dental Association Council on Dental Therapeutics; you'll find it on the carton or tube of those fluoride toothpastes the association considers proved effective.

Now, for the proper brushing technique, hold the brush sideways against your teeth with the bristles at a forty-five-degree angle facing into the gum. Wiggle the head of the brush back and forth with almost circular strokes, while the bristles—pushed into the crevices where gums meet teeth—remain nearly stationary; only the tips of the bristles get in just under the gums to loosen the plaque. You can clean the cheek and tongue sides of all your teeth this way, two at a time. To clean the tongue side of your front teeth, brush with the "toe," or front part, of the brush, and use the same wiggling motion with short up-and-down strokes. Next brush the inside of the back teeth and the chewing surfaces with short back-and-forth strokes, and wind up by brushing the rough upper surface of your tongue where debris and bacteria also tend to collect and produce bad breath.

Between flossing and brushing this is going to take you anywhere from fifteen to twenty minutes, but when you consider that periodontal treatment can eat up a half year of your time and a couple of thousand dollars, it's well worth it.

BAD BREATH

Television commercials for various mouthwashes have been compelled to abandon claims of killing germs that cause bad breath—tantamount to the claims that toothpastes and powders can whiten teeth. The FDA no longer permits mouthwash manufacturers to claim their products have any therapeutic value as regards halitosis. The most any mouthwash can do is temporarily freshen your breath, but again, that's no small accomplishment. No bright smile, after all, should be wedded to a sour breath, and happily, nine times out of ten bad breath can be easily remedied.

Mouthwashes come in a variety of flavors and colors, but should yours ever run dry, try a mix of baking soda and water. It may not give you the psychological lift of, say, a cinnamon-flavored mouthwash, but it works. A sprig of parsley is another foe of halitosis; that explains why so many upper-mobile hamburger-and-onion emporiums station a bowl of cracked ice and parsley alongside the register for departing customers. (Furthermore, parsley's known as the "wonder leaf" with twice as much iron as spinach and three times as much vitamin C as oranges.) Finally, make it a daily habit to brush your tongue every time you brush your teeth; it's still one more way to fight bad breath.

YELLOW TEETH

Smoking and coffee, tea, and cola drinking all stain teeth. So if you've been smoking, say, since high school, your teeth probably advertise the fact. Then, of course, some yellowness is inherited. But if you have discolored teeth, take heart, for there's a new treatment available which some dentists are now using for patients with exceptionally dingy-looking teeth. The whole surface of the tooth is covered with a paste called composite resin. There's no drilling, no shot of novocaine. It's painless, but it isn't exactly a bargain. The front upper six teeth, for example, can be done in two hours at a cost of about $500 to $600.

DRY, CHAPPED LIPS

While dry, chapped lips are certainly not aesthetically offensive, they do nothing to enhance a man's appearance, and they tend to be associated with aging, despite the fact that a teenager can have them if he's exposed to too much sun, wind, or extreme cold. Lip dehydration's no problem, however; get yourself a stick of clear, oil-based lip gloss (Chapstick is one such product), and apply it several times daily, or use a stick coated with cooling camphor (Chesebrough-Pond's has one called Vaseline Camphor Ice that works fine for both chapped lips and hands).

COSMETIC DENTISTRY

Tooth jacketing is the most common cosmetic procedure performed by dentists. It's a reasonably simple procedure that's painless, thanks to mild sedation and a high-speed technique, but unless your teeth are really misshapen, I can't see cutting into perfectly good teeth simply to cover the resultant shell with a whiter, brighter model. Today, however, most dentists leave a good portion of the tooth intact. The procedure goes like this.

Something like a ledge is drilled in the tooth, under the gum, over which the jacket, or crown, is forced and locked into place, guaranteeing protection of the natural tooth and security of the jacket or crown. A temporary crown is worn before the permanent one is cemented into place.

The usual flossing technique won't work with a jacketed tooth. Your dentist will show you how by inserting an open-end plastic toothpicklike dart, you can slip the floss between the jacketed tooth and its neighboring teeth on either side.

MISSING TEETH

When I was growing up, it wasn't at all uncommon for a man of forty to have false teeth top and bottom. Not so today, of course, what with better diet and regular visits to the dentist. Still, sometimes a tooth must be pulled, and when it is, replace it without delay. Open spaces can throw not only the bite off but sometimes the entire jaw out of line, and it can even impair hearing, all because of stress' being placed in the wrong places. Teeth, after all, should fit together like meshing gears, and when they don't, stress results. Pressure exerted by the jaws can be as much as 300 pounds per square inch, so to keep and maintain a healthy mouth and a winning smile, replace missing teeth as soon as possible.

Part Two

LOOKING...
AND *FEELING*
LIKE A MILLION

How to Conquer Stress

A healthy body and a more placid frame of mind are the ticket to feeling like a million. The proper diet and the right kind of exercise done regularly will provide a healthy, good-looking body. But more difficult to achieve is the placid frame of mind. Must we pay with our mental health for the tensions of our modern world? No, not if we learn what causes emotional wear and tear and how to minimize them in our daily lives.

A certain amount of stress is essential to good, robust living. It stimulates that extra flush of adrenaline to energize body and brain just when we need it most. It's when stress gets out of hand, when it takes over and has you squirming on the end of the line that you're in trouble—often big trouble.

Medical statistics suggest that 50 to 80 percent of present-day diseases have their origins in stress, and most doctors believe that almost every disease is aggravated by stress. Dr. Robert Giller, a New York internist with a master's degree in nutrition, says, "Stress makes any illness worse—from the common cold to a broken arm."

Dr. John Prutting, who has written extensively on the subject of stress, describes it this way: "Medically and biologically, stress is a state in which a chain of glandular and hormonal reactions takes place to help the body adapt to its physical and emotional environment. . . . But when these adjustment demands on the body are extreme, or continual, the body's adaptive mechanisms may break down, and you can become ill—even die."

No man today is exempt from periods of extreme emotional stress. I'm sorry to report that it is estimated that 10 percent of American men now age forty-five won't make it to fifty-five, and stress-related diseases are a contributory cause. There's substantial evidence that high blood pressure, heart attacks, strokes—perhaps even cancer—may be the result of the body's inability to cope with stress, while ulcers (an estimated 8 million Americans have ulcers), and severe headaches (there are approximately 12 million migraine headache sufferers) can be directly or indirectly traced to stress.

On still another level, an ineffectual response to stress can lower self-esteem, cause depression, scramble the ability to concentrate and make decisions, and blunt the sex drive and ability to perform. But it is entirely possible to cope effectively and healthfully with stress in your life without resorting to pills or booze. (One more depressing statistic, and I'll lay off: It's estimated that 14 percent of all men take Valium.)

SYMPTOMS

No two men react the same to stress. One man may start taking naps during the day, while another suffers from insomnia. One man loses his appetite, and the other stuffs himself between meals. But here are the most common symptoms of stress gone out of control:

> Rapid heartbeat
> Tensing of muscles in arms and legs
> Stiff neck
> Grinding of teeth
> Shortness of breath
> Excessive perspiration

STRESS IN WASHINGTON, D.C.

In the spring of 1979 I was in Washington and fortunate enough to attend "Health Works '79," a three-day extravaganza created by the Department of Health, Education, and Welfare with cooperation from the President's Council on Physical Fitness and Sports and the National Park Service. There were circuslike tents fluttering flags and offering films and live exhibitions; small armies of teenagers out on the grass beside the Mall performing rhythmic gymnastics; and senior citizens doing aerobic dancing on an outdoor stage. There was also a slide cartoon program devoted to understanding and coping with stress as well as a quiet area serving as a place to relax and refresh. So far as stress goes, here's what I gained in knowledge from that visit.

1. Physical exercise can relax you and help you deal with mental and physical stress; moderate exercise is a first-rate stress reliever. Combine stretching with deep breathing, for example. Reach for the sky, then for your toes; breathe deeply a few times; then reach again slowly, letting your muscles stretch while your body releases the tension.

2. Learn to accept what you can't change.

3. Balance work and recreation. Schedule time for recreation to relax your mind.

4. Take one thing at a time. It's defeating to tackle all your tasks at once; instead, set aside some of your time, and work on the more urgent.

5. The absence of work is not necessarily a way to avoid stress. Work is actually good for you as long as you can achieve something and feel successful by doing it.

6. Make a list of the people you would turn to in a crisis. Don't underestimate the importance of having someone to talk to.

7. Get enough sleep. It's refreshing. Lack of sleep can lessen your ability to deal with stress by making you more irritable.

8. Eating a balanced diet is a giant step toward helping your body cope with stress.

LEARN TO RELAX

Dr. Norman Orentreich says, "If you have inner equanimity, it helps everything." But how do you achieve it? Some men find it in yoga and Tai-Chi, the ancient Hindu and Chinese exercise philosophies. Yoga's stretching and breathing exercises have a massaging effect on the nerves, while the lesser-known Tai-Chi movement exercises—slow, coordinated, natural, and easy—are designed to bring body and mind into a condition of equilibrium.

Some corporations encourage their hardworking executives to take up transcendental meditation. The august *Wall Street Journal* in August 1972 devoted a front-page article to it as a technique for relaxation:

> Thousands of otherwise conservative businessmen, scientists, teachers and housewives have taken up the practice, reporting such beneficial effects as freedom from tension, mental wellbeing and heightened energy and creativity. Although skeptics abound, they seem to be far outnumbered by converts and true believers. And, lending a new respectability to the practice are doctors and researchers at universities and hospitals.

Dr. Herbert Benson, of the faculty of the Harvard University Medical School, tested a group of meditators and found that during meditation their blood pressure was low and their heart and respiration were slowed—measurable physiological effects that are the direct opposite of stress.

As I wrote earlier, moderate exercise is a first-rate stress reliever. Brisk walking, for example, acts like a tranquilizer for jangled nerves. Dr. John Prutting, prominent New York internist, believes that "for the control of the emotions, there is no exercise better than walking," thus echoing Dr. Paul Dudley White, the famed cardiologist of the Eisenhower era, who maintained, "A vigorous five-mile walk will do more good for an unhappy but otherwise healthy adult than all the medicine and psychology in the world."

How? According to Dr. Edward Greenwood of the Menninger Clinic in Topeka, Kansas, "The physical stimulation induces an intellectual stimulation through the central nervous system. The ego is strengthened, accompanied by a greater feeling of self-confidence, stability, and calmness."

THE SAUNA

Its champions claim that the sauna cleanses the body of toxins, increases resistance to colds, helps you shed poundage, and improves circulation. Its detractors, on the other hand, say that's overstating the case. On the subject of the sauna, Dr. Charles Kuntzleman, national program consultant of the YMCA Fitness Finders Program in Spring Arbor, Michigan, flatly states, "The only demonstrated therapeutic claim is relaxation it may produce if used correctly."

The Finns invented the sauna and know how to enjoy it, and I had my first sauna in Helsinki more than a decade ago: dry heat up to 200° F, skin slapping with birch branches, buckets of cold water, and vigorous massage, followed by a plunge in the snow outside. I don't know whether the experience cleansed my body of toxins, but I felt great afterward—wonderfully relaxed. Too many Americans enter a sauna already exhausted and dehydrated by rigorous exercise. Then the sauna makes them sweat even more, robbing their bodies of fluids to the point of heat exhaustion. Furthermore, the high heat can aggravate a heart condition because the body must struggle to maintain normal temperature.

But if you think a sauna will help you cope with stress—and I think it might—bear in mind the following guidelines devised by Dr. Kuntzleman:

1. Keep temperature at or below 185° F and the humidity at 10 percent or lower. (The drier the air, the more easily sweat evaporates.)

2. Wear as little clothing as possible—to facilitate the evaporation of sweat.

3. Spend no more than eight to ten minutes in the sauna the first time.

4. Don't stay in the sauna alone. Heat stroke can sneak up on you.

5. After a large meal, wait at least one to two hours before using the sauna.

6. Never use the sauna if you're under the influence of alcohol or drugs—including antihistamines.

WILL YOUR BODY TO RELAX

You can learn. It takes practice, but eventually the ability to relax at will can become a part of your living routine.

1. Take off your shoes, loosen your belt and tie, and stretch out on a bed or sofa, arms at your sides. The most important thing is that you be physically comfortable in a quiet, calm environment. Tell yourself that in ten to twenty minutes you're going to get up feeling completely relaxed. (If you think you might relax to the point of dozing off, sit in a chair instead. The idea is that you stay awake throughout this relaxation exercise, remaining in complete control.)

2. Now close your eyes, and breathing through your nose slowly, begin a body inventory, starting with your feet. As you concentrate on each body part, try to visualize the tension there melting away.

3. As you concentrate on your feet, wiggle your toes as though you were shaking the tension off.

4. Concentrate next on your entire leg, clear up to the hip. Think of each leg growing more and more relaxed. It might help to picture the tension as a coil of ectoplasm leaving the leg and vanishing in midair.

5. Think about your arms, from your fingertips to your elbows and then all the way up to your shoulders. Spread your fingers, and feel the tension passing down and out through them.

6. Think of your stomach, and breathe more deeply. Imagine the muscles there have been knotted, and now, with each breath you inhale and exhale, those knots unravel until all tension has gone. Signal the final release from tension with a deep sigh of relief.

7. Continue breathing deeply as you think of your chest and neck. Part your lips slightly, and imagine the tension slipping through them and away from you.

8. Your neck is now so relaxed that it feels almost limp. Let the relaxed feeling move up into your face. Open your mouth, drop your jaw, and feel the tension start to slip away from the muscles there and out through your mouth. Eyes closed, imagine that your entire body is becoming so relaxed that you feel as though you were floating a few feet above where you're lying. Say to yourself, "I am deeply, completely relaxed." Wiggle your toes; flex your ankles; spread your fingers wide; open your mouth and yawn. Breathe in and out, smoothly and evenly, and feel how relaxed and refreshed every part of you has become.

9. Take a deep breath, exhale, and open your eyes. Slowly sit up, get to your feet, stretch both arms over your head, and then slowly lower them to your sides. Stand tall; feel proud. You've just conquered stress. Relaxation is a learned skill, and now that you've learned it, it's going to become a habit with you.

Eating Well

Awareness is the first step in learning to modify and control what you eat. Dr. Judith Rodin of Yale University deplores what she calls the diet mentality because she feels that "a diet takes control away from the individual and you stop learning": learning the facts about the foods your body needs to stay well; learning the basics of nutrition, which is nothing more than how you interact with your food.

At least 70 million Americans are overweight, according to Dr. Victor Herbert, a physician and professor of medicine at the State University of New York, who concludes, "The major nutritional problem in the country is obesity." Elsewhere it's been called our food-abundant nation's number one malnutrition problem, for despite the fact that we spend an estimated 20 percent of our income for food, many of us are what nutritionists call weight-control illiterates, nutrition ignoramuses.

Fad diets with fat-burning tricks have practically become a cottage industry. But the problem of obesity isn't simply to lose weight, but to keep weight off, and most diets are so strict, so self-punishing that people just won't stick to them. Inevitably, they regain whatever weight they lose because the diet doesn't permanently modify their eating behavior.

The only way to get fit and stay fit is to learn something about nutrition. Dr. Nevin Scrimshaw, head of the Department of Nutrition and Food Science at MIT, says, "The human body does not adapt well to obesity. Maintaining normal body weight is not a cultural or aesthetic choice. It, along with a well-balanced diet, is the basis of good health." And good nutrition, like exercise, isn't a sometime thing. It means a well-balanced diet, and that in turn means a variety of good foods—a lifelong, day-to-day good habit.

ARE YOU OVERWEIGHT?

If you can't answer that by looking in a mirror, reach over to the skin overlying the side of your chest, and pinch; if there's more than an inch of skin between your fingers, you're probably overweight. Still, a scale is by far the simplest and most efficient gauge of over-

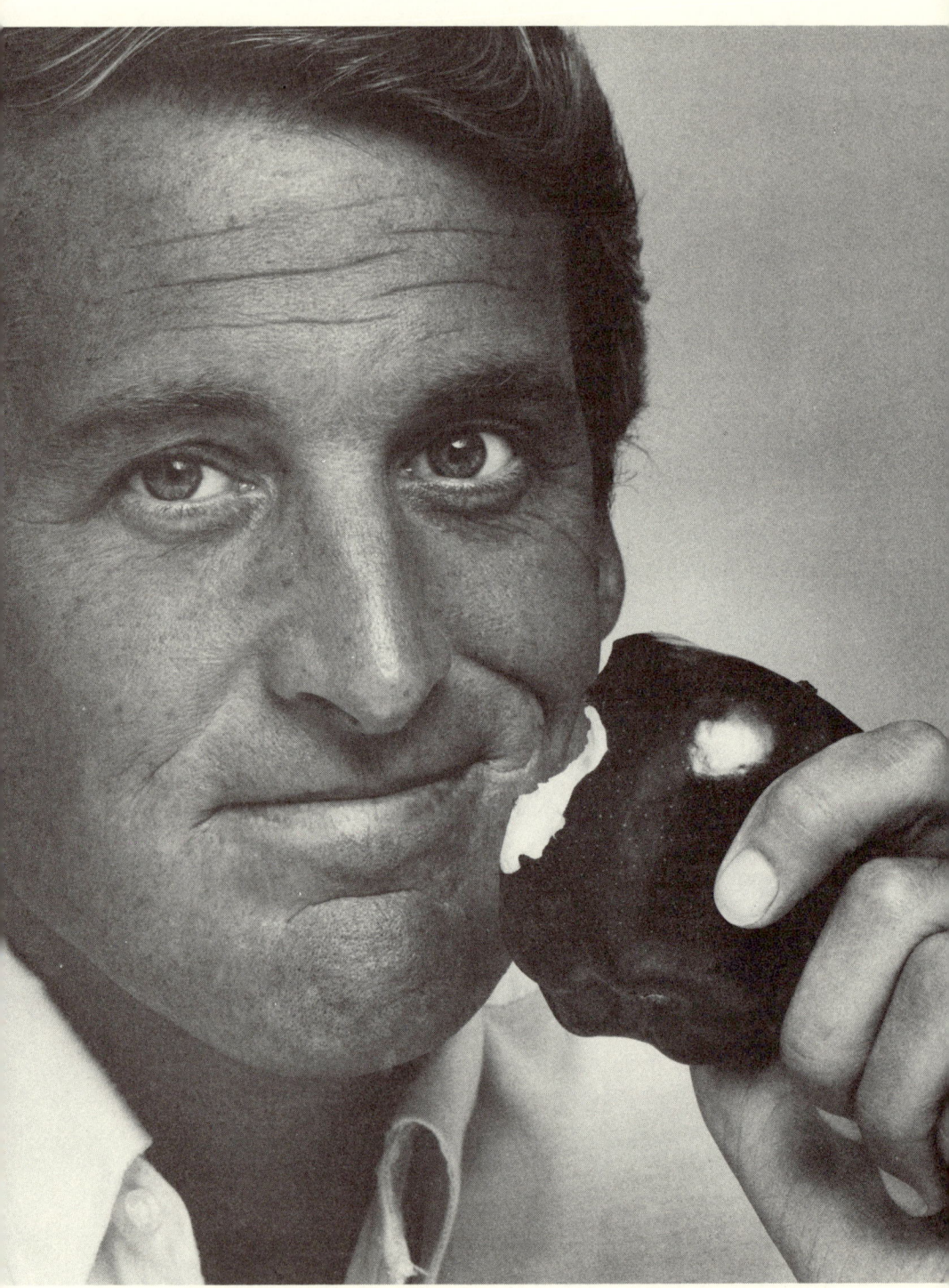

PHOTO BY ROBERT EPSTEIN.

eating. Weigh yourself at the same time of day with little or no clothing once a week or, better yet, every day, and you'll soon know whether your calorie intake has been too high, too low, or the proper amount to maintain normal body weight.

Do you remember how much you weighed at age twenty-five? That's considered a man's ideal weight, provided, of course, his weight was normal at the time. Every year over age twenty, you need ten calories less per day to maintain your weight.

The following are the height and weight standards for adult males (in indoor clothing *) given by the Metropolitan Life Insurance Company. Since no two men are built exactly alike, I don't think there's such a thing as an ideal weight for a given height. So let this table merely serve as a guide. You may look and feel your best a few pounds more or less than the range indicated for your height and frame.

Feet	Inches	*Small Frame*	*Medium Frame*	*Large Frame*
5	1	112–120	118–129	126–141
5	2	115–123	121–133	129–144
5	3	118–126	124–136	132–148
5	4	121–129	127–139	135–152
5	5	124–133	130–143	138–156
5	6	128–137	134–147	142–161
5	7	132–141	138–152	147–166
5	8	136–145	142–156	151–170
5	9	140–150	146–160	155–174
5	10	144–154	150–165	159–179
5	11	148–158	154–170	164–184
6	0	152–162	158–175	168–189
6	1	156–167	162–180	173–194
6	2	160–171	167–185	178–199
6	3	164–175	172–190	182–204

SLIMMING DOWN

How do you go about it? Start at the very beginning, and learn to accept these basic truths: When it comes to losing weight, there

* Allow 5–7 pounds

are no tricks, no shortcuts. A calorie is still a calorie no matter what its source, and the only way you can get rid of fat is to burn it up as fuel; otherwise, it is stored.

Nutritionist Adelle Davis, whose books have outsold everything between covers except the Bible, had a nifty guide for sensible eating: Breakfast like a king, lunch like a prince, and dine like a pauper. In short, the later the day, the fewer calories you should consume for the good reason that you have less time, less opportunity to burn them up. I think it's a good rule to consume two-thirds of your day's calories by 2:00 P.M.

The choice as to what you eat and how much is yours because you can do more for your health than any doctor or any hospital can.

Should you need motivation, consider this: After forty-five, it's indicated that for people ten pounds overweight there is an 8 percent increase in the death rate; twenty pounds overweight, 18 percent; thirty pounds overweight, 28 percent; and fifty pounds overweight, 56 percent. "The smaller your waistline, the longer your lifeline," is how it is put by world-renowned nutritionist Gayelord Hauser, who, at eighty-four, stands six feet three and weighs a svelte 185 pounds.

Many Americans consume 3,300 calories a day (approximately 50 percent more than the recommended daily allowance), and about 40 to 45 percent of those calories are in the form of fat; in short, almost half of what we eat is *fat*. While some fat is needed in the diet, Dr. Richard Rivlin, chief of nutrition at the Cornell University Medical College, believes that the basic needs of the body can be met with a much lower fat content. Most other leading authorities agree, suggesting that a 25 percent fat diet provides enough fat for the body's energy to run smoothly. But Nathan Pritikin, founder-director of the Longevity Center in Southern California, known in some circles as the Lourdes of the West for people suffering from medical problems ranging from angina and hypertension to arthritis and diabetes, has created the now-famous Pritikin Diet, which cuts down fat consumption to a mere 5 to 10 percent.

The fat factor is our big nutritional concern today on two levels: (1) Fat is high in calories because ounce for ounce, fat supplies more calories than either protein or carbohydrates; and (2) overweight is perhaps *the* American disease. Fat, especially saturated fat, is linked to cardiovascular disease, the nation's number one killer with more than one-fourth of its victims men between the ages of forty-five and sixty-five. Dr. Rivlin advises eliminating the foods that are very high in fat, especially the saturated kind found in rich cheeses, pastries, ice cream, and red meat.

Red meat was once considered macho, the ticket for energy and endurance. "We are the only country I think of which has male and female foods," says Dr. Jean Mayer, nutritionist and president of Tufts University. "Women eat chicken croquettes, but for the man it's a big slab of rare meat. It's the motorcycle of the middle-aged, the last refuge of macho." It's estimated that each one of us consumes 193 pounds of red meat a year, much of it riddled with cholesterol.

We all carry cholesterol in our bodies, manufacturing it in our intestinal tracts and livers. In the right amount, this waxy, fatlike substance helps us maintain healthy bodies, but if we take in too much of it via the foods we eat, as we age it becomes embedded in the lining of the artery walls, and eventually the arteries narrow and may block the flow of blood to that part of the body. If that occurs in a major artery serving the heart, the result is a coronary; if it's in the brain or a vessel leading to the brain, the result is a stroke. So cut down on your intake of cholesterol-rich foods. Eat no more than three egg yolks a week. Choose lean cuts of meat, trim all visible fat, and discard the fat that cooks out of the meat; better yet, eat more fish and chicken. Avoid deep-fat frying. Instead of whole milk and cheeses made from whole milk and cream, use skim milk and skim milk cheeses. Instead of butter and other cooking fats that are solid or completely hydrogenated, use liquid vegetable oils and margarines that are rich in polyunsaturated fats.

Follow those rules, and you'll cut down not only on fat but on calories, too. Compare: Two ounces of white meat of chicken or turkey contain 100 calories, while rib roast of beef (not trimmed of fat) contains 250 calories. A half pint of skim milk contains 80 calories, while a half pint of whole milk has 150 calories.

The American Heart Association * recommends six basic food groups, the number and size of servings for each, and then what foods in these six groups either to avoid or to use sparingly.

1. MEAT, POULTRY, FISH, DRIED BEANS, AND PEAS, NUTS, EGGS

   1 serving. . . .

   3–4 ounces of cooked meat or fish (not including bone or

---

* © Reprinted with permission of American Heart Association.

fat) or 3–4 ounces of a vegetable listed here. Use 2 or more servings (a total of 6–8 ounces) daily.

Recommended

Chicken, turkey, veal or fish in most of your meat meals for the week.

Shellfish: clams, crab, lobster, oysters, scallops and shrimp are low in fat but high in cholesterol. Use a 4-ounce serving as a substitute for meat no more than twice a week.

Beef, lamb, pork and ham less frequently.

Choose lean ground meat and lean cuts of meat. Trim all visible fat before cooking. Bake, broil, roast, or stew so that you can discard the fat which cooks out of the meat.

Nuts and dried beans and peas:

Kidney beans, lima beans, baked beans, lentils, split peas and chick peas (garbanzos) are high in vegetable protein and may be used in place of meat occasionally.

Egg whites as desired.

Avoid or Use Sparingly

Duck and goose.

Heavily marbled and fatty meats, spare ribs, mutton, frankfurters, sausages, fatty hamburgers, bacon and luncheon meats.

Organ meats—liver, kidney, heart and sweetbreads—are very high in cholesterol. Since liver is very rich in vitamins and iron, it should not be eliminated from the diet completely. Use a 4-ounce serving in a meat meal no more than once a week.

Egg yolks: limit to 3 per week, including eggs used in cooking.

Cakes, batters, sauces and other foods containing egg yolks.

2. BREAD AND CEREALS (Whole grain, enriched or restored)

1 serving . . . of bread:

1 slice

1 serving . . . of cereal:

½ cup cooked
1 cup, cold, with skimmed milk
Use at least 4 servings daily.

Recommended

Breads made with a minimum of saturated fat:

White enriched (including raisin bread), whole wheat, English muffins, French bread, Italian bread, oatmeal bread, pumpernickel and rye bread.

Biscuits, muffins and griddle cakes made at home, using an allowed liquid oil as shortening.

Cereal (hot and cold), rice, melba toast, matzo, pretzels.

Pasta: macaroni, noodles (except egg noodles) and spaghetti.

Avoid or Use Sparingly

Butter rolls, commercial biscuits, muffins, donuts, sweet rolls, cakes, crackers, egg bread, cheese bread and commercial mixes containing dried eggs and whole milk.

3. VEGETABLES AND FRUIT (Fresh, frozen or canned)

1 serving: ½ cup
Use at least 4 servings daily.

Recommended

One serving should be a source of Vitamin C:

Broccoli, cabbage (raw), tomatoes, berries, cantaloupe, grapefruit (or juice), mango, melon, orange (or juice), papaya, strawberries, tangerines.

One serving should be a source of Vitamin A—dark green leafy or yellow vegetables, or yellow fruits:

Broccoli, carrots, chard, chicory, escarole, greens (beet, collard, dandelion, mustard, turnip), kale, peas, rutabagas, spinach, string beans, sweet potatoes and yams, watercress, winter squash, yellow corn. Apricots, cantaloupe, mango, papaya.

Other vegetables and fruits are also very nutritious; they should be eaten in salads, main dishes, snacks and desserts, in addition to the recommended daily allowances of high Vitamin A and C vegetables and fruits.

Avoid or Use Sparingly

If you must limit your calories, use vegetables such as potatoes, corn or lima beans sparingly. To add variety to your diet, one serving (½ cup) of any of these may be substituted for one serving of bread or cereals.

4. Milk Products
1 serving. . . .
8 ounces (1 cup)

Buy only skimmed milk that has been fortified with Vitamins A and D. *Daily servings:* Children up to 12—3 or more cups; Teenagers—4 or more cups; Adults—2 or more cups.

Recommended

Milk products that are low in dairy fats:

Fortified skimmed (non-fat) milk and fortified skimmed milk powder and low-fat milk. The label on the container should show that the milk is fortified with Vitamins A and D. The word "fortified" alone is not enough.

Buttermilk made from skimmed milk, yogurt made from skimmed milk, canned, evaporated, skimmed milk and cocoa made with low-fat milk.

Cheeses made from skimmed or partially skimmed milk, such as cottage cheese, creamed or uncreamed (uncreamed, preferably), farmer's, baker's, or hoop cheese, mozzarella and sapsago cheeses.

Avoid or Use Sparingly

Whole milk and whole milk products:

Chocolate milk, canned whole milk, ice cream, all creams including sour, half and half, whipped, and whole milk yogurt.

Non-dairy cream substitutes (usually contain coconut oil, which is very high in saturated fat).

Cheeses made from cream or whole milk.

Butter.

5. Fats and Oils (Polyunsaturated)

An individual allowance should include about 2–4 tablespoons daily (depending on how many calories you can afford) in the form of margarine, salad dressing and shortening.

Recommended

Margarines, liquid oil shortenings, salad dressings and mayonnaise containing any of these polyunsaturated vegetable oils: Corn oil, cottonseed oil, safflower oil, sesame seed oil, soya-bean oil and sunflower seed oil.

Margarines and other products high in polyunsaturates can usually be identified by their label which lists a recommended liquid vegetable oil as the first ingredient, and one or more partially hydrogenated vegetable oils as additional ingredients.

Diet margarines are low in calories because they are low in fat. Therefore it takes twice as much diet margarine to supply the polyunsaturates contained in a recommended margarine.

Avoid or Use Sparingly

Solid fats and shortenings: Butter, lard, salt pork fat, meat fat, completely hydrogenated margarines and vegetable shortenings and products containing coconut oil.

Peanut oil and olive oil may be used occasionally for flavor, but they are low in polyunsaturates and do not take the place of the recommended oils.

6. Desserts, Beverages, Snacks, Condiments

The foods on this list are acceptable because they are low in saturated fat and cholesterol. If you have eaten your daily allowance from the first five lists, however, these foods will be in excess of your nutritional needs, and many of them also may exceed your calorie limits for maintaining a desirable weight. If you must limit your calories, limit your portions of the foods on this list as well.

Moderation should be observed especially in the use of alcoholic drinks, ice milk, sherbet, sweets and bottled drinks.

Acceptable

Low in calories or no calories: Fresh fruit and fruit canned without sugar, tea, coffee (no cream), cocoa powder, water ices, gelatin, fruit whip, puddings made with non-fat milk, low calorie drinks, vinegar, mustard, ketchup, herbs and spices.

High in calories: Frozen or canned fruit with sugar added, jelly, jam, marmalade, honey, pure sugar candy such as gum drops, hard candy, mint patties (not chocolate), imitation ice cream made with safflower oil, cakes, pies, cookies and puddings made with polyunsaturated fat in place of solid shortening, angel food cake, nuts, especially walnuts, peanut butter, bottled drinks, fruit drinks, ice milk, sherbet, wine, beer and whiskey.

Avoid or Use Sparingly

Coconut and coconut oil, commercial cakes, pies, cookies and mixes, frozen cream pies, commercially fried foods such as potato chips and other deep-fried snacks, whole milk puddings, chocolate pudding (high in cocoa butter and therefore high in saturated fat) and ice cream.

THE WELL-BALANCED DIET

The body takes its fuel from food, and because the body's energy requirements diminish with age, we should eat less as we grow older. Rather than the 3,300 calories a day most of us consume, Dr. Rivlin suggests that a diet of 2,500 calories a day is adequate for an adult male. But often what we *don't* eat is as important as what we eat. And what we need to stay well and energetic has been established by the Nutrition Board of the National Academy of Science and is known as RDA (Recommended Daily Allowances).

Vitamin	*RDA*	*Sources*
A	5,000 IU *	Green and yellow fruits and vegetables, milk, dairy products, fish-liver oils. A cup of cooked spinach gives 8,000 IU; one raw carrot, 10,000 IU; one whole tomato, 1,250 IU.
B_1	1–1.5 mg †	Brewers' yeast, brown rice, blackstrap molasses, wheat germ, peanuts, poultry, nuts. 1¼ cups of peanuts provide 1 mg; 4 tablespoons of brewers' yeast, 2.25 mg.
B_2	1.3–1.7 mg	Blackstrap molasses, whole grains, nuts, organ meats. 2 slices of beef liver provide 2 mg.
B_6	1.5–1.8 mg	Blackstrap molasses, brewers' yeast, leafy green vegetables, organ meats, wheat germ, egg yolk, and milk. Would you believe that only 1 cup of peas provides 2 mg?

* International Units
† Milligrams

Vitamin	RDA	Sources
B_{12}	3 mcg*	Milk, dairy products, fish, organ meats. A single egg contains 1 mcg; a ½-lb. can of tuna, 5 mcg.
B_{15}	None given	Whole grains, brown rice, organ meats.
C	45 mg	Fresh citrus fruits, vegetable juices, cantaloupe, red and green peppers. One green pepper gives 120 mg; one orange, one grapefruit, 100 mg each.
D	400 IU	Sunshine, cod-liver oil, egg yolk, organ meats. A ¼-lb. can of tuna or salmon has 300 IU.
E	12–15 IU	Eggs, organ meats, wheat germ, vegetable oils, green lettuce, avocados. Two tomatoes, 3 IU; one tablespoon of safflower oil, 20 IU.

Mineral	RDA	Sources
Calcium	800–1,400 mg	Milk, buttermilk, cheese, yogurt, powdered skim milk, molasses. One slice of American cheese provides 200 mg.
Iodine	100–130 mcg	Seafood, iodized salt, kelp tablets. One kelp tablet is purported to provide 150 percent of the RDA.
Iron	10–18 mg	Liver, apricots, oysters, organ meats, blackstrap molasses, eggs, wheat germ. A ¼-lb. serving of beef liver gives 200 mg.
Magnesium	300–350 mg	Honey, nuts, seafood, spinach, bran. One cup of roasted peanuts, with skin intact, provides 420 mg.

* Micrograms

Mineral	RDA	Sources
Phosphorus	800 mg	Meat, poultry, fish, egg yolk, peas, beans, grains, yogurt. A ¼-lb. serving of calf's liver, 600 mg.
Potassium	None given	Raisins, peanuts, seafood, dates, figs, peaches, blackstrap molasses, baked potato. One whole banana, 500 mg; one baked potato, 500 mg.
Zinc	15 mg	Brewer's yeast, spinach, liver, mushrooms, seafood.

While most of us nowadays are fairly knowledgeable about vitamins, we probably fall into the "nutrition ignoramuses" class when it comes to minerals, a pity, too, since the body can tolerate a deficiency of vitamins for a longer period of time than it can a deficiency of minerals.

Dr. John Prutting, the New York internist who has made a study of nutrition, considers magnesium "the miracle mineral that keeps you fit . . . the 'control mineral' that keeps the body." Unfortunately magnesium levels in the body lessen as we grow older. Poor diet and heavy drinking are the commonest causes of magnesium deficiency (alcohol depletes body magnesium). Dr. Prutting estimates that 70 percent of us have mismanaged our diets enough to have some degree of magnesium deficiency, and chronic deficiency can contribute to hardening of the arteries. Check out your diet, and determine if you're "magnesium poor." Along with spinach, other particularly rich sources of this important mineral are broccoli, brussels sprouts, and kale. When you prepare vegetables, I suggest you steam instead of boil them; steaming does not leach out the nutrients the way boiling does. A stainless steel vegetable steamer basket costs under $4 and fits any pot.

Space doctor Charles Berry, a NASA consultant and medical director of the Houstonian, an eighteen-acre $30 million medical center for businessmen, has prescribed potassium to stop the irregular heartbeats some astronauts experience in space.

Now a final word on the well-balanced diet—the essential fuel for efficient body performance. Dr. Frederick Stare of the Harvard School of Public Health says that it is one that includes fruits and vegetables, cereals, some milk, and small servings of lean meat, chicken, and fish—in short, a diet that concentrates on canny nutrition, not deprivation or excess. *Any* food taken in excess can be harmful.

CONSTIPATION

Can diet cause constipation? It certainly can. Eating the wrong foods or eating too little can cause constipation. Elimination—cleansing the body—is easier, more natural if your diet contains some roughage. Whole grain breads and cereals, such as barley, brown rice, oats, and wheat, and green leafy vegetables are good sources of roughage. Bran is probably the single most important dietary factor which prevents constipation; it isn't a laxative but rather a regulator of bowel function. When you take bran, it's advisable to begin with one or two teaspoons a day, increasing the amount until you feel it's working best for you.

If constipation becomes a problem, also concentrate on cellulose-rich foods, such as figs, dates, apples, nuts, raw tomatoes, and cantaloupes.

As for laxatives, I suggest that you see your doctor before buying one of the "natural" over-the-counter laxatives. Most of them tend to cause dependence on them for bowel movement, and that's to be avoided. Also, some of them come under the category of the stimulant or irritant laxative. They work by irritating the nerves of the colon and that way stimulating it to contract, and taken over a prolonged period of time, they damage the nerves within the wall of the colon, sometimes permanently.

THE MEGAVITAMIN CONTROVERSY

The term "megavitamin" translates to the use of massive doses of vitamins. If vitamins spell good health, can more vitamins mean SUPERhealth?

Some doctors maintain that if we eat all the varieties of food good nutritionists recommend on a consistent basis, we don't need vitamin supplements. (One large carrot, for example, will provide the daily requirement of vitamin A, and huge excesses of this vitamin over a period of time can slowly make you pretty sick.) Other doctors believe that taking vitamins is relative and conditional, that individual needs for vitamins vary widely, and that some individuals need larger amounts than the recommended daily allowance (RDA). I know of one well-known television personality who totes a popcorn bag of vitamins wherever he goes. Every day some 86 million Americans take vitamin pills, many of them so-called natural vitamins, which means organically grown. They're no more beneficial than the synthetic ones; they just cost more.

What it all boils down to is this: Vitamin-taking has become highly controversial—to the point that the Food and Drug Administration has decreed vitamins containing more than 150 percent of the recommended daily allowance must be classified as drugs.

In the opinion of Dr. Frederick Stare, "The greatest harm with megavitamin therapy is that the patient puts off seeking competent medical advice that can usually take care of his problem." On the other hand, Dr. Elizabeth Whelan, executive director of the American Council on Science and Health, regards megavitamin therapy as "the latest shortcut to good health. . . . It can do harm in at least two ways: High doses of some vitamins are health-threatening (A and D), and possibly high doses of C can be harmful," while Dr. Victor Herbert believes that megadoses of vitamin C may actually block the action of vitamin B_{12}, which is important to a healthy nervous system.

Whether you need vitamin pills as a dietary supplement is something to be decided by you and a physician—one who has a working knowledge of nutrition. Unfortunately physicians like that are not yet in great supply.

CUT DOWN ON SUGAR

The average American consumes nearly 120 pounds of sugar a year. Sugar consumption in the United States has doubled since the turn of the century, and many physicians equate the rise with the dramatic 500 percent increase in coronary heart disease over the past fifty years. A report in the Swiss medical journal *Praxis* on March 9, 1971, noted that Swiss heart disease death statistics for the years 1900 to 1968 parallel Switzerland's increased sugar consumption.

The "Seven Commandments" of the Pritikin Diet read: "Thou shalt not smoke, nor eat fats, sugar, salt nor foods containing excess cholesterol; neither shalt thou drink coffee or tea." But doesn't sugar provide quick energy? It does, but quick energy is soon lost, leaving you feeling worse off than before.

Furthermore, sugar has been refined to a degree that it's been devitalized, adding calories to your diet but nothing in the way of vitamins and minerals. MIT nutritionist Warren M. Navia told a meeting of the American Chemical Society back in 1972, "The increased consumption of sugar and sugar products threatens our nutritional balance."

Enough said.

RETIRE YOUR SALT SHAKER

The average American consumes four or five teaspoons of salt a day, a total of fifteen pounds a year. We so overdose ourselves with salt that the Center for Science in the Public Interest, a nutrition advocacy group, has asked the Food and Drug Administration to begin regulating the substance in processed foods and labeling foods for their salt content. Much of the salt we eat is hidden in foods not thought of as salty: canned soups, packaged breakfast cereals, bread, puddings, pancakes, and almost all commercially canned vegetables. Canned asparagus, for example, contains fifty times more salt than fresh asparagus.

Why this sudden emergence of salt as a dietary villain? Well, it is now thought to be a major precipitating cause of hypertension, which afflicts some 25 million Americans. Worldwide surveys have found that people who don't eat much salt have little or no sign of hypertension. The Lenox Hill Hospital's Hypertension Center in New York City advises: "If you are overweight, if you use a lot of salt, or both, you should realize that you are neglecting two factors that adversely affect blood pressure. . . . To put it in simple terms, lower your weight and salt intake and you lower the risk of high blood pressure."

All the sodium your body needs—and more—is already there in the foods you eat. You don't need to add salt, it's a habit you should break. Dr. Robert M. Giller, a New York physician who specializes in nutrition, says, "The average person in the United States consumes at least ten times more salt than the body requires."

Cut down on salty foods. Use fresh vegetables instead of canned; if you do use canned vegetables, drain off the liquid, and heat them in tap water. Use unsalted butter and margarine. There are even a few brands of club soda that are labeled salt-free. Salt, after all, isn't the only seasoning; try onions, scallions, garlic, chives. Better yet, go light on the seasoning altogether, and discover the hidden flavor in your foods.

THE RISE OF THE NUTRITIONIST

Eating under the guidance of a nutritionist is sometimes called programmed eating. But just *who* is a nutritionist?

Classically a nutritionist is a medical doctor with a master's degree in nutrition. All people who call themselves nutritionists, however, are not of this classic mold. Some are dietitians, and others are Ph.D.'s and self-styled practitioners.

Dr. Giller considers himself "an old-time doctor." Nutritional education, he says, is only part of his practice. "I also emphasize the importance of exercise and relaxation." He thinks that too many people tend to departmentalize their well-being. "Some come to me and say, 'Give me some vitamins.' Because nutrition has become so popular, people look to it as a panacea. They think if they eat right, all problems will disappear. This is not to diminish the importance of a good diet, but I want to stress that a patient may have other problems that are not nutrition-related—problems that may require a complete life-style change."

Today increasing numbers of affluent men see two practitioners: a medical doctor and a nutritionist. It's still a rare doctor who knows much about nutrition, and medical schools are only just now adding nutrition courses to their curricula. Senator Richard Schweiker of Pennsylvania, who has been on both the Health Committee and the Select Committee on Nutrition and Human Needs, has long urged that all medical schools set up nutrition education programs, and Dr. Jean Mayer of Tufts University firmly believes that no one should be allowed to graduate from high school without having had a solid course in nutrition. "Good eating habits make for healthy people," he says.

There are almost as many theories and approaches to diet as there are nutritionists. Dr. Richard S. Rivlin explains, "The information we have is not conclusive." Still, he feels that a competent nutritionist should be capable of explaining the nutritional composition of foods, outlining a good eating plan, and advising whether certain eating habits and food additives are harmful or not.

Most nutritionists aim at adapting special diets to the patient's life-style and emotional makeup. Dr. Giller, for instance, says he helps "evolve a good eating program for an individual," which involves two visits to his office. From conversation during the first visit, Dr. Giller gets to know something of the patient's life-style and, as a result of the patient's history and a physical examination, gives him a tentative diet to follow. At a second visit one month later the patient reports on his progress, and by that time all laboratory tests (blood test, hair analysis,* urinalysis, computerized analysis of the diet, and so on) are back. On the basis of their findings, Dr. Giller makes any necessary adjustments in the patient's eating plan and prescribes the necessary vitamins and minerals. "Rather than an out-and-out diet—most diets are so awful I try to show the individual how to restructure his diet—I make it very simple. First, eliminate the foods that are bad for the general population—those we know are the main causes of disease. In short, I cut down on fats and refined carbohydrates. And I watch out for food additives. I test for the patient's hidden food allergies and then determine which vitamins and minerals are needed."

Despite the fact that controversy abounds in the field of nutrition, more and more men whose careers demand high energy and the ability to cope with constant stress are seeking the advice of nutritionists. And you don't hit upon a proper diet and then set it and forget it because our nutritional needs change as we change. But one thing does remain constant: Every nutritionist I've talked to agrees that you shouldn't eat anything if you don't recognize the ingredients listed on the label. "Read the labels," they all urge.

* Hair is a living chronicle of your body's mineral content, and modern testing techniques can detect possible overloads or shortages of minerals.

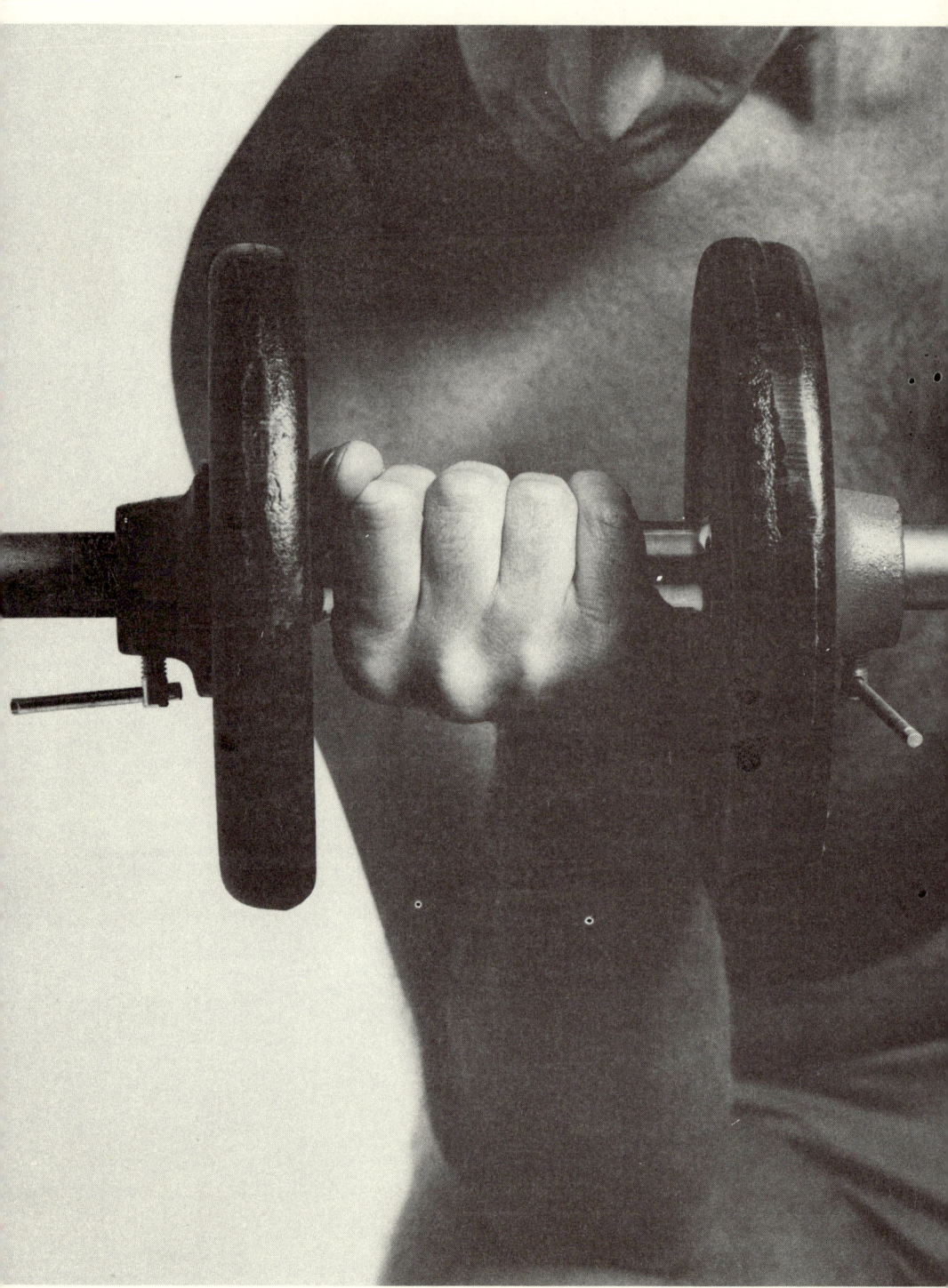

PHOTO BY ROBERT EPSTEIN.

Exercising Regularly

In its fullest sense, fitness is an integrated system which involves your body, mind, and soul. It is a state of health, of looking and feeling good. It helps keep your figure trim and your posture right, and it minimizes fatigue. It helps your body respond to unusual demands and ward off disease. It is the way to a longer and healthier life.

—Dr. James A. Nicholas, founder and director of the Institute of Sports Medicine and Athletic Trauma at Lenox Hill Hospital in New York City

Dr. Nicholas takes care of the New York Jets, New York Knicks, New York Rangers, New York Cosmos, and New York Yankees, so he's speaking from firsthand experience. He promotes fitness as an integral part of a man's daily life.

Happily, we're into a physical fitness boom, which is attributed to several things—increased leisure time, shapelier body-conscious clothing, and, as one magazine writer put it, "Perhaps the most significant reason . . . the masses have finally discovered what athletes have known all along. That exercise makes you feel good." To be fit is to be happy.

Dr. Irving Dardik, chairman of the Sports Medicine Committee of the U.S. Olympic Committee and a leading vascular surgeon, defines exercise as "the science of movement." Moving your body around and making all your muscles work—regularly—that's what dynamic health is all about. The body has more than 500 muscles, but in his daily routine, the average man probably uses about 8 percent of his.

Well, it's never too late to start exercising. Senator William Proxmire, a self-described physical fitness buff, maintains that if you exercise regularly and vigorously, eat a moderate and balanced diet, and learn how to relax, you can be in far better shape as you get older than when you were young. "When I say you can be in better shape in maturity—in your forties, fifties, sixties—than you were between fifteen and twenty-five, which is considered the prime of physical life, it is based on my own experience. If you exercise enough, you will be leaner, stronger, more energetic."

Speaking at a "Fitness After Fifty" conference sponsored by the Center for the Study of Aging held at the Institute on Man and Science in Rensselaerville, New York, Dr. Herbert deVries, director of the Exercise Physiology Laboratory at the University of Southern California, told of setting up a mobile research facility at Laguna Hills Leisure World where he gathered 112 nonathletic men aged fifty to eighty-seven, gave them physical examinations, tested reactions, then put them through hour-long workouts three times a week. After a six-week period of calisthenics, jogging, stretching, and water exercises, Dr. deVries repeated all the pre-exercise tests and then compared his new physical culturists with another group of eight nonexercising men. The results were astonishing. The exercisers averaged a 5 percent drop in body fat, a 6 percent reduction in diastolic blood pressure, a 9 percent rise in maximum oxygen consumption, and a 7.2 percent increase in the strength of their arms. It was further revealed that the men who exercised had cut nervous tension by as much as 23 percent!

Older men who exercise vigorously have less than one-third the incidence of heart attack of men who don't exercise. Seventy-three-year-old Paul Fairbanks of Washington, D.C., ran six and a half miles per hour for two and a half hours on a treadmill that was part of a float in President Jimmy Carter's inaugural parade. And Fairbanks didn't start a running program until he was sixty-three.

Should you have a physical checkup before starting an exercise regimen? Yes, but Dr. Samuel M. Fox III, a member of the President's Council on Physical Fitness and Sports, addressing a group of physicians, said that a physical checkup is more urgent for those who plan to remain inactive than for those who intend to get into good physical shape.

Dr. David Stonecypher, fellow member of the American Geriatrics Society, says, "When an older person rests, he rusts." In fact, we start getting rusty after age thirty, the chief problem being the emphasis our schools give to team sports. Except for men's track and swimming, the major sports in high school and college are team-oriented. Nothing is done to motivate anybody to exercise when there's no longer a team and a coach around, and to compound the problem, the team-oriented man who stops regular exercise once he leaves school still maintains the same eating habits he had when he was physically active and really burning up the calories. Overeating and a sedentary life-style bring on flabbiness, overweight, chronic low-back pain, weak abdominal muscles, high pulse rate, shortness of breath, and increased susceptibility to hypertension and coronary heart disease. Our overfed, underexercised society has the highest coronary death rate in the world. But regular vigorous exercise can delay this decline. The human body is a machine, and like any machine, it's built for action, and it will break down if you don't use it. Energy initiates energy; inactivity leads to deterioration. Eat well, exercise regularly, and you'll soon be able to determine the food-exercise ratio that will keep you fit and healthy.

Dr. Hans Kraus, clinical associate professor of physical medicine and rehabilitation at the New York University Medical School, maintains that the physically inactive individual shows signs of aging earlier in life and is "less well equipped to meet the daily stresses of life than the active person." The Committee on Aging of the American Medical Association agrees, endorsing regular exercise as a potent defense against "deterioration" on the basis of a ten-year study. Regular exercise can change your level of fitness to that of a man ten to twenty years younger.

All this should provide any man with enough motivation to get moving, but Dr. Dardik believes that to have an effective exercise routine, you need understanding along with motivation because getting—and staying—in shape requires a routine developed for a man's individual requirements, capacities, and temperament; fitness takes time, thought, and consistency. Find the exercise routine that's right for you—one that's comfortable and pleasurable—and you'll stay with it. Otherwise, without the natural high of pure enjoyment, you'll probably find good reasons to stop. According to Dr. Dardik, "We should have fun while we exercise, as children do in active play, and make it a natural part of our lives."

Keep your exercise routine safe and simple. The idea that exercise has to involve a lot of straining and sweating is passé. Dr. David Costill, director of the Human Performance Laboratory at Ball State University in Indiana, says, "If you can't talk while you're exercising, you're working too hard." It's not a matter of the more exercise, the better, but of finding the right kind of exercise for you.

Alexander Mallaby, YMCA fitness expert, cautions that "a chosen sport should not be so competitive that it turns into a field of battle." Your sport should help release tension, not create it.

HOW MUCH EXERCISE IS ENOUGH?

About fifteen minutes a day, three times a week is the minimum exercise prescription given by one of the nation's leading cardiologists. Three exercise sessions per week proved more effective than five sessions per week for a group of adult males in Canada. A study at the University of Western Ontario compared the results of forty exercise periods in twenty-four subjects. Half the group exercised three times a week; the other half, five times a week. The researchers found that participants who exercised fewer times each week, but over an extended period of time, gained the highest fitness level.

But doesn't exercise stimulate the appetite? The answer is no. Actually, when an inactive person decides to start exercising, his appetite is not stimulated—it's reduced. No one knows why for sure, but after about twenty years of research it's accepted as fact. Some researchers think it's probably due to a shift in hormone balance, said to be a natural reaction when an individual switches from a sedentary life to an active life. Air Force Major Bruce S. Harger, a physician who does physical education research, says, "We note changes in appetite in the cadets who join us at the Air Force Academy each year. One of the factors for their curbed appetite is an increase in exercise."

A 1978 nationwide survey revealed that business leaders are much more likely than the general public to participate in some kind of regular exercise activities. Many blue-chip corporations today equate good health with good business, for men who exercise regularly are found to be more assertive, show their aggressions more readily, and have greater emotional stability than non-exercisers. That is undoubtedly why an increasing number of giant corporations are providing their executives with fully equipped gymnasiums for on-the-job workouts. Yet the majority of the leadership surveyed still felt that they weren't getting enough exercise, and one of the main reasons given was a lack of interest. That takes us back to the point made earlier: Whatever exercise program you choose should become a comfortable, pleasurable habit; if it is, there'll be no lack of interest.

THE BEST KIND OF EXERCISE

The best is the one that keeps you on the move and raises your heartbeat to about 70 percent of its maximum attainable rate. To calculate your MHR—the highest number of beats per minute of which your heart is capable—simply subtract your age from 220 to get a reasonably accurate estimate.

Maximal Heart Rate by Age

Age	MHR	70 percent of maximum
20	200	140
30	190	133
40	180	126
50	170	119
60	160	112
70	150	105
80	140	98

It's important that you count your pulse rate, which is almost always the same as the number of heartbeats per minute, *immediately* upon stopping exercise. Find the beat within a second, and count for ten seconds; then multiply by six to obtain the count for a minute. (Take your pulse by using the first two or three fingers on the outside of the wrist of the opposite hand.)

According to Dr. Paul Dudley White, the famed cardiologist, "The only sports that improve physical fitness are those that encourage rhythmical, continuous, nonsensitive exertion involving leg muscles"—in other words, aerobic or endurance exercise. Jogging, walking, swimming, bicycling (Dr. White was riding his bike around Boston when well past his seventieth birthday), cross-country skiing, and rope jumping all are aerobic exercises that allow the maximum amount of oxygen to be delivered to the blood, lungs, and heart. ("Aerobic" means "with oxygen.") It's interesting to note that most cardiologists today favor brisk walking over jogging for achieving and maintaining physical fitness, believing that while jogging is certainly an excellent conditioner, it's best suited for men under forty.

A year-round sport is a wise choice, and most of the aerobic exercises fill that bill. You can, after all, swim outdoors in summer and at indoor pools in winter and walk any season of the year. Of course, you can substitute one seasonal sport for another, but you may use your body differently for each sport. The transition, as a result, may have to be made slowly, and you may lose something in the process.

RATING FOURTEEN SPORTS AND EXERCISES FOR PHYSICAL FITNESS

The following scoreboard offers a summary of how seven medical experts rated fourteen different sports and exercises in promoting physical fitness. The ratings are on a scale of 0 to 3; thus, a rating of 21 (rated 3 by seven judges) is the maximum score.

	Jogging	Bicycling	Swimming	Skating	Handball/Squash	Skiing-Nordic	Skiing-Alpine	Basketball	Tennis	Calisthenics	Walking	Golf (using caddie)	Softball	Bowling
Physical Fitness														
Cardiorespiratory endurance (stamina)	21	19	21	18	19	19	16	19	16	10	13	8	6	5
Muscular endurance	20	18	20	17	18	19	18	17	16	13	14	8	8	5
Muscular strength	17	16	14	15	15	15	15	15	14	16	11	9	7	5
Flexibility	9	9	15	13	16	14	14	13	14	19	7	8	9	7
Balance	17	18	12	20	17	16	21	16	16	15	8	8	7	6
General Well-Being														
Weight control	21	20	15	17	19	17	15	19	16	12	13	6	7	5
Muscle definition	14	15	14	14	11	12	14	13	13	18	11	6	5	5
Digestion	13	12	13	11	13	12	9	10	12	11	11	7	8	7
Sleep	16	15	16	15	12	15	12	12	11	12	14	6	7	6
Total	148	142	140	140	140	139	134	134	128	126	102	66	64	51

Note: Ratings for golf are based on the fact that many men use a golf cart or caddie. Playing golf that way has prompted one leading nutritionist to comment, "Golf burns up as many calories as playing the cello."

But if you walk the links, the physical fitness value moves up appreciably. George Romney, former Michigan governor and secretary of HUD, tees off, then runs to pick up the ball. In short, he jogs between shots.

SOME OPINIONS ON
OTHER SPORTS AND EXERCISES

About volleyball, canoeing, water-skiing, and horseback riding, Dr. Samuel Fox, Professor of Medicine, Georgetown University, says:

"Volleyball is less demanding than basketball and can be easier to organize teams with odd numbers and less equal skills than with basketball. A good mix of exertion and sociability.

"Canoeing is good total body exercise if done vigorously as in stream or whitewater paddling (with associated hazards).

"Water-skiing is good fun but noisy, and needs expensive equipment. Largely isometric, with anxiety component which makes it not good for heart disease patients.

"Horseback riding provides good exercise but is expensive and there is some hazard."

Dr. Lawrence E. Lamb, syndicated medical columnist, points out that ". . . unless they are included in calisthenics, we have omitted real strength-type exercises, such as muscle training or weight training, from our consideration. That is a mistake because developing good strong muscles is part of maintaining good posture, which is important to health as well as appearance."

About team sports, Dr. Hans Kraus, an orthopedic physician, says: "For school-years fitness, team sports and any other sports should come second to fitness-creating activities which include jogging, running, and calisthenics for basic minimum muscular fitness. Team sports are most likely to back-fire and give only the most fit a chance to compete, leaving on the sidelines the ones who need activity the most."

And Dr. Evalyn S. Gendel of the Kansas University Medical School points out that "fitness activities of a team or group often cannot be guaranteed to continue throughout life. Also, sometimes anxiety issues related to team activities cause digestive, nervous or distractive influences affecting sleep, etc."

Dr. Gendel also regretted that the panel had not considered dancing and gymnastics: "Since fitness and sports concerns both sexes, I was sorry to see dancing (modern, ballet, folk and free form) plus gymnastics omitted from the list. These activities offer a great deal of exertion for both men and women. Their benefits are again universal for activity, alone or in groups, and also add the element of music for its psychological as well as physical input."

THE MOST UNDERRATED EXERCISES

Rope skipping is considered by some to be the perfect exercise, reducing fat on legs, thighs, and hips, improving the sense of balance, increasing agility, and adding strength to the muscles all over the body. It's claimed that 500 hops in five minutes, three or four times a week, will maintain a satisfactory level of fitness. You need no special equipment other than a length of sash cord, no special clothing, and it can be done anywhere. It has long been a conditioning exercise for the in-training prizefighter, and exercise physiologist Jack Baker, head of the Human Performance Laboratory of Murray State University in Kentucky, has conducted experiments demonstrating that about the same level of fitness is achieved within ten minutes of skipping as in thirty minutes of jogging.

The stationary bike has made a comeback. For years it was largely dismissed as boring—practically a nonexercise. It may still spell boredom to some men, but for others it's a safe, sane way to provide a good heart/lung workout and lose weight in the bargain. There's only one hitch: You must cycle for a half hour every day.

Walking, man's first really good habit, is finally being given the acclaim it deserves. Dr. Grant Gwinup, chairman of the Department of Metabolism and Endocrinology at the University of California, calls it "the one exercise that does everything."

We were born to walk. Walk briskly, and literally every part of your body performs naturally—muscles stretch and turn and knead with every step, and lungs dilate with air. Furthermore, it's a risk-free exercise you can stay with for your entire life.

Never ride when you can walk. Start walking to work, or get off the train one stop early. Skip the elevator; use the stairs instead. Senator William Proxmire walks the five miles from his office to his home every night and considers it "a marvelously well-spent hour."

I don't suggest that walking should be your only form of exercise, but I do think that it should be your basic exercise. It will improve your coordination, breathing, and stamina and make you more proficient at whatever sport you choose.

THE GYM DANDY

Johnny Carson's home gymnasium is filled with gleaming steel devices, pulleys and springs and counterweights. The so-called core of actor Clint Eastwood's body building is two one-hour daily workouts in an elaborate home gym, where, among things, he hoists a twenty-pound dumbbell plate behind his head and does parallel-bar dips for his arms and chest. Weight lifting is all right, says Dr. Willibald Nagler, physiatrist-in-chief at New York hospital, so long as you don't press weights *over* your head; that, he says, puts too much stress on the spine. According to Dr. Nagler, at about twenty-five or thirty, the disks that cushion the vertebrae start to thin out, and further stress only accelerates this process. Result: the chance of a slipped disk or the bones pressing on nerves and causing a lot of back pain. So lift weights if you want, but skip overhead weight lifting.

THE EXERCISE STUDIO

You'll find no weight lifting equipment here, for the whole idea is to build lean, well-toned muscles rather than bulging Arnold Schwarzenegger types of muscles. A plus on the side of the exercise studio is that joining an exercise class helps commit you to a regular schedule.

The fourteen Nickolaus Exercise Centers in New York City, Philadelphia, Beverly Hills, and Richmond, Virginia, offer a prime example of this exercise genre. The Nickolaus Technique, as it's called, consists of a series of thirty exercises done in a set sequence with each group of movements utilizing its own breathing pattern. All-over body conditioning is the goal, with almost all the exercising done on the floor, using the body as the resistance rather than working against the forces of gravity via heavy equipment. Still, this is vigorous exercise with special emphasis on straightening and strengthening the spine while toughening the abdominal muscles and lower back—the two most commonly troublesome weak spots for the over-forty crowd.

Dance exercise studios, meantime, are mushrooming across the country. Their exercises are excellent all-around muscle toners as well as a guaranteed way to correct the posture habits that lead to bad backs, tension, and fatigue. In fact, many of the stretching exercises so popular today are spin-offs, if not exact copies, of the limbering-up exercises the dancer does at the ballet barre. And ballet is a terrific sport; in fact, all forms of dancing (ballet, modern, folk, and free-form) offer a great deal of exertion for a man.

TRAVEL FITNESS

Again and again many of the men I talked to while working on this book complained that frequent business travel made it difficult for them to exercise regularly. Granted, but with some planning and the proper budgeting of time, you can do it no matter how often or how far you travel. You'll not only feel better and look better for doing it but also think more sharply when the time comes to sit down and talk business.

Let's say that running is part of your regular exercise regimen. Allow yourself an hour in the morning so that you can run before breakfast. In fact, early-morning running is so popular with traveling executives these days that many hotels provide guests with the best jogging routes within a mile or so radius of their location. And first-thing-in-the-morning brisk walking requires even less preparation since there's not an ounce of special gear required.

As already noted, all you need for rope skipping is a length of sash cord. It takes up precious little space in your luggage, and you can get in your hops in the privacy of your hotel room.

Practically all first-classs hotels and motels nowadays have swimming pools, so why book into one that doesn't?

You see, there's really no excuse for not exercising while traveling. In fact, I think it's vitally important that the business traveler —inevitably subject to a certain amount of stress what with making planes, meetings, and weighty decisions—should make a point of exercising every day no matter where in the world he happens to be.

THE HEALTH SPA

This is a total environment: a program of exercise, regulated diet, body massage, and such extras as being wrapped, mummylike, in a cocoon of steaming-hot herbal-soaked sheets. It's a hedonistic experience, an escape from reality, and a *super*vacation that a friend swears everyone should experience at least once in his lifetime.

The most plush health spas seem to flourish in California, Florida, and Mexico, where a one week's stay can run anywhere from a low of $600 to well over $1,500.

To give you some idea of what life's like at a health spa, here is the schedule at the Golden Door in Escondido, California:

5:30–6:30 A.M.: a five-mile mountain climb or straight three-mile walk, followed by weighing in; sauna; steam bath or shower.

7:30 A.M.: breakfast.

8:30–9:00 A.M.: warm-up exercises.

9:00–10:00 A.M.: class with stretching, strengthening, endurance exercises.

10:00–11:00 A.M.: gym with special emphasis on strengthening.

11:00–Noon: water exercises.

Noon: massage.

1:00 P.M.: lunch.

2:00 P.M.: volleyball in pool.

3:00 P.M.: jogging, afternoon walk, gym, or swimming.

4:00 P.M.: break for afternoon snack.

5:00–6:00 P.M.: stretch and relax class.

6:00–6:30 P.M.: change for dinner.

6:30 P.M.: cocktails.

7:00 P.M.: dinner, followed by a brisk walk.

8:00 P.M.: lectures or movies or just talking.

The only possible drawback to a week or two at a health spa is that after you have surrendered your body and will to a staff of experts for renewal and rejuvenation, there's sometimes no incentive to keep up the good work once you're back in the real world and left to your own devices.

THE FOUNTAIN OF YOUTH

Recent research suggests that a vigorous program of swimming may counteract the normal effects of aging. Most of us see only about 40 percent of our breathing level, but a good swim forces breathing, so gives the body deep, full ventilation. That is why you experience a sense of euphoria after a good swim. A regular swimming program, furthermore, will improve heart, arteries, and lungs, lower blood pressure, and reduce the concentration of cholesterol in the blood. There are psychological benefits as well; studies suggest that swimmers are more sexually active and have a more positive self-image, greater concentration, less anxiety, and a greater sense of control over their lives than nonswimmers.

Senator Jacob Javits of New York, in his seventies, swims in the Senate pool every day Congress is in session. Harry Helmsley, perhaps the nation's premier landlord, with real estate holdings stretching from New York to San Francisco conservatively valued at some $3 billion, swims a quarter of a mile daily in his pool atop his two-story penthouse overlooking New York's Central Park. Past seventy, Helmsley is trim and vital, with the energy of a professional athlete half his age.

Aqua Dynamics is the name given to a program of physical conditioning through water exercises developed by the President's Council on Physical Fitness and Sports. A person immersed to the neck in water experiences an apparent weight loss of 90 percent of his weight; as a result, people usually find it comfortable to exercise in the water. The following Aqua Dynamics can be done in a small pool or in a limited area of a large, crowded pool.*

Warming Up

During a workout the body should be warmed up by light conditioning and stretching exercises before heavier activities are attempted. Deck exercises including flexibility and strength activities with heavy breathing are appropriate. Various strokes may be simulated. Participants should begin with light rhythmical work at a slow pace. A tempo should be gradually accelerated, alternating slow with faster work, until one nears perspiration.

Most swimming activities cause the back to be in hyperextended position, thus specific back stretching exercises should be completed both at the beginning and end of the workout. For maximum benefit, the individual should stand with legs apart, extending the hands high over head and reaching as high as is possible. After approximately 5–10 seconds in the arms-over-head reaching position, one should bend the trunk forward and down, flexing the knees, and the bending and

---

* Reprinted with permission of the President's Council on Physical Fitness and Sports.

stretching position should be held for approximately 20–30 seconds, then the high reaching followed by the bending and stretching action should be repeated.

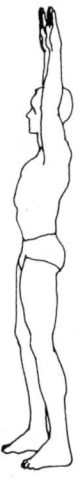

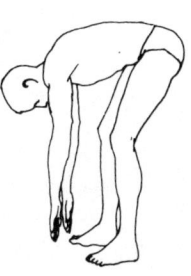

Through proper warm-up the body's deep muscle temperature will be raised and the ligaments and connecting tissues stretched, thereby preparing the body for vigorous work. This will help avoid injury and discomfort.

The following is Aqua Dynamics, a regimen of high-potential physical activities which can be used in a small pool or in a limited area of a crowded institutional pool.

STANDING WATER DRILLS

Alternate Toe Touch

Standing, in waist-to-chest deep water, swimmer:

(1) Raises left leg bringing right hand toward left foot looking back and left hand extended rearward.
(2) Recover to starting position. Repeat. Reverse.

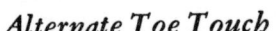

Side Straddle Hop

Standing in waist-to-chest deep water with hands on hips, swimmer:

(1) Jumps sideward to position with feet approximately two feet apart.
(2) Recovers.

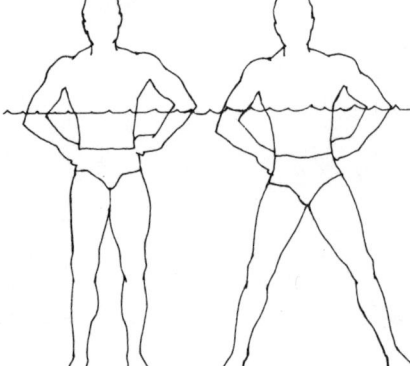

Stride Hop

Standing in waist-to-chest deep water with hands on hips, swimmer:

(1) Jumps, with left leg forward and right leg back.
(2) Jumps, changing to right leg forward and left leg back. Repeat.

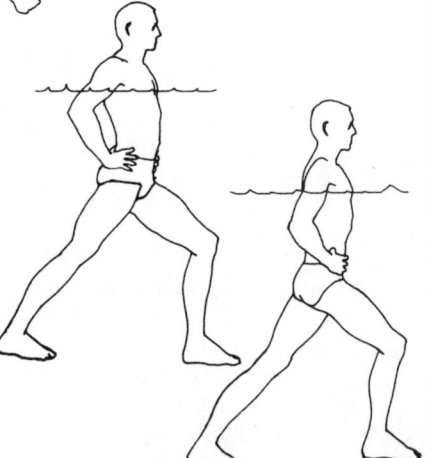

Toe Bounce

Standing in waist-to-chest deep water with hands on hips, swimmer:

(1) Jumps high with feet together through a bouncing movement of the feet.
Repeat.

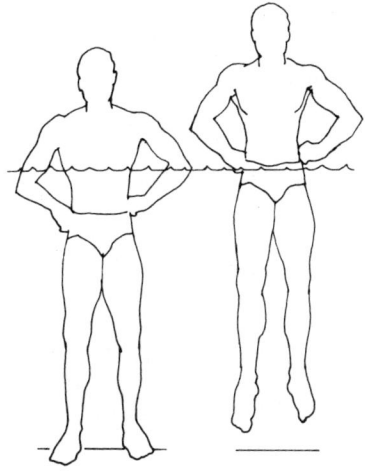

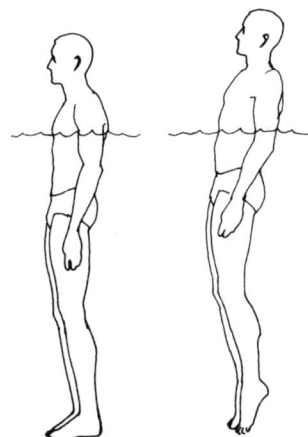

Raise on Toes

Standing in chest-deep water, swimmer:

(1) Raises on toes.
(2) Lowers to starting position.
Repeat.
Accelerate.

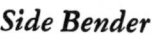

Side Bender

Standing in waist-deep water with left arm at side and right arm over head, swimmer:

(1) Stretches, slowly bending to the left.
(2) Recovers to the starting position.
Repeat.
Reverse to right arm at side and left arm overhead.

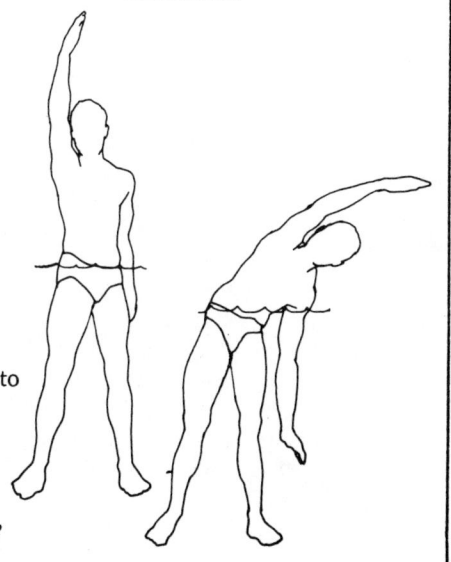

Standing Crawl

Standing in waist-to-chest deep water, swimmer:

(1) Simulates the overhand crawl stroke by:
  (a) Reaching out with the left hand, getting a grip on the water, pressing downward and pulling, bringing the left hand through to the thigh.
  (b) Reaching out with the right hand, etc.
  Repeat.

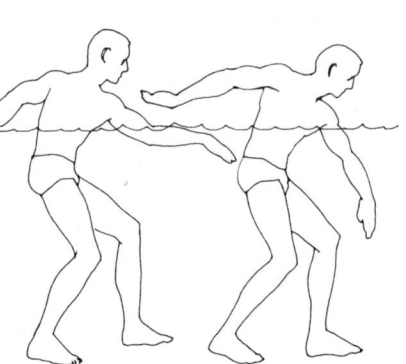

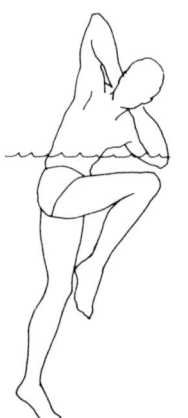 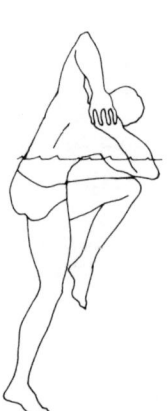

Walking Twists

With fingers laced behind neck, swimmer:

(1) Walks forward bringing up alternate legs twisting body to touch knee with opposite elbow.
Repeat.

Bouncing

Standing in chest-deep water, swimmer:

(1) Bounces on left foot at the same time pushing down vigorously with both hands causing the upper body to rise, and
(2) Bounces similarly on right foot pushing down with both hands, etc.
Repeat.

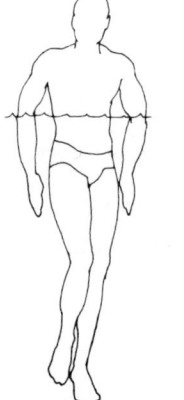 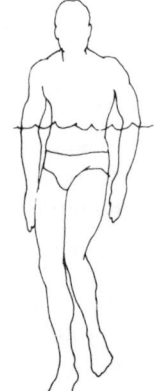

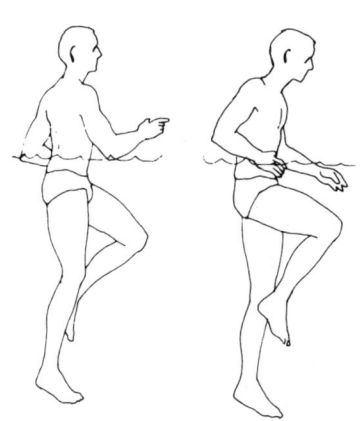

Jogging in Place

Standing with arms bent in running position, swimmer:

(1) Jogs in place.

GUTTER-HOLDING DRILLS

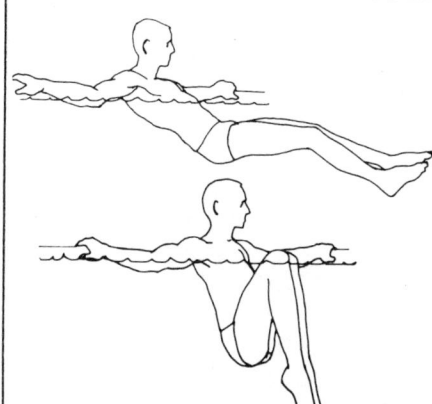

Pool-side Knees Up

Supine, holding on to pool gutter with hands and legs extended, swimmer:
(1)   Brings knees to chin.
(2)   Recovers to the starting position.
Repeat.

Twisting Legs

Supine, holding on to pool gutter with legs extended, swimmer:

(1)   Twists slowly to left.
(2)   Recovers.
(3)   Twists slowly to right.
(4)   Recovers.
Repeat.

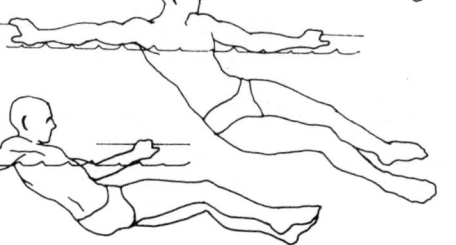

Knees Up Twisting

Supine, holding on to pool gutter with knees drawn up to chest, swimmer:

(1) Twists slowly to left.
(2) Recovers.
(3) Twists slowly to right.
(4) Recovers.
Repeat.

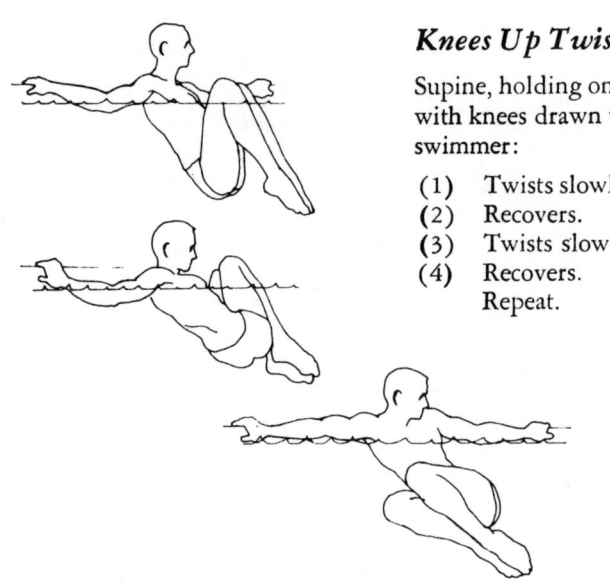

Leg Crosses

Supine, holding on to pool gutter with legs extended, swimmer:

(1) Swings legs far apart.
(2) Brings legs together crossing left leg over right.
(3) Swings legs far apart.
(4) Brings legs together crossing right leg over left.
Repeat.

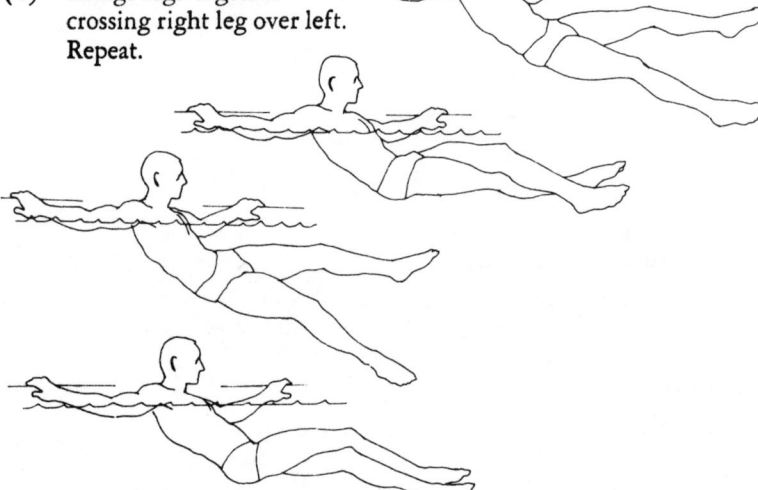

Alternate Raised Knee Crossovers

Standing, holding on to pool gutter with hands, back to wall:

(1) Lifts left knee and crosses it over. Twists to the right.
(2) Recovers.
(3) Lifts right knee and crosses it over, twisting to left.
(4) Recovers.

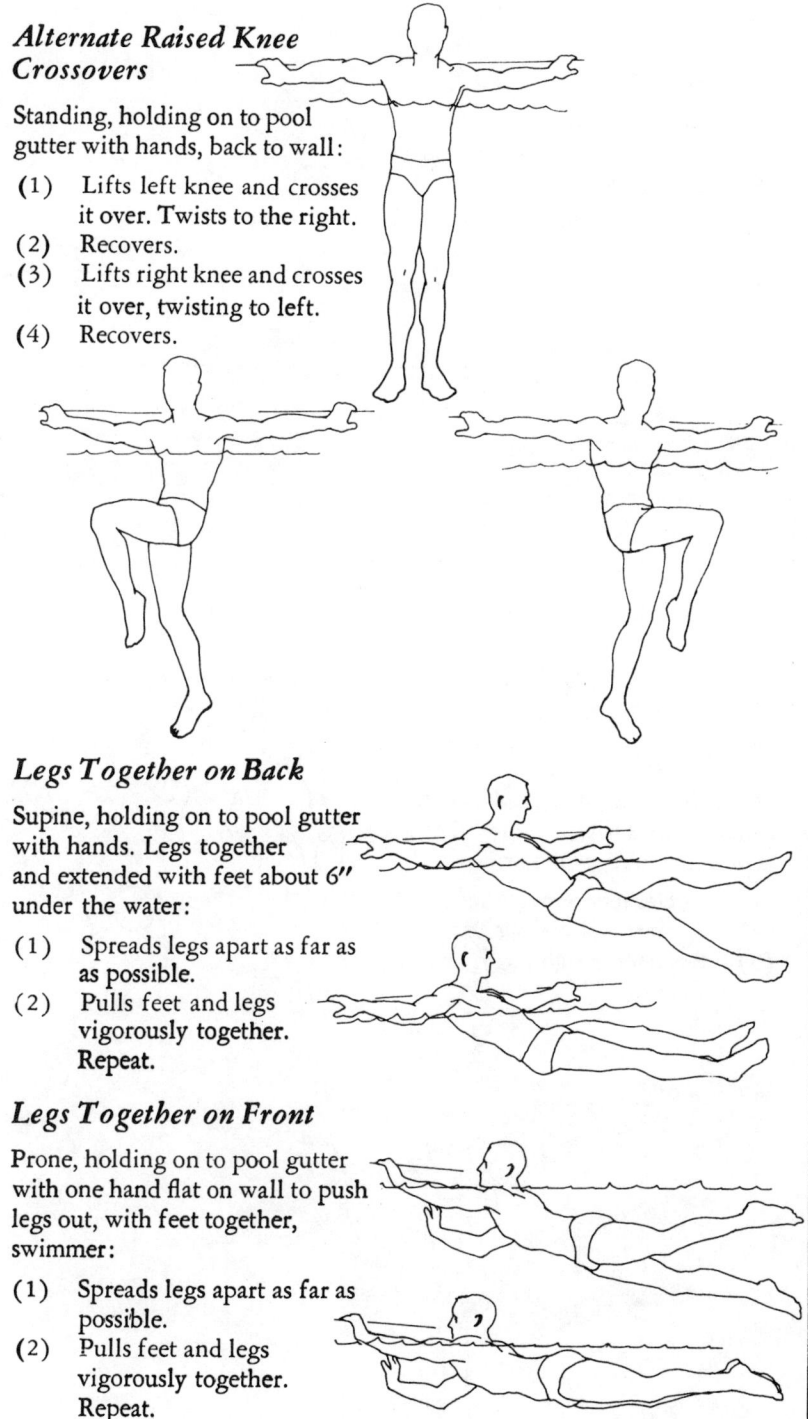

Legs Together on Back

Supine, holding on to pool gutter with hands. Legs together and extended with feet about 6" under the water:

(1) Spreads legs apart as far as as possible.
(2) Pulls feet and legs vigorously together. Repeat.

Legs Together on Front

Prone, holding on to pool gutter with one hand flat on wall to push legs out, with feet together, swimmer:

(1) Spreads legs apart as far as possible.
(2) Pulls feet and legs vigorously together. Repeat.

Raising Hips

Prone, holding on to pool gutter with one hand flat on wall to push legs out, swimmer:

(1) Raises hips, holding for four counts.
(2) Relaxes.
   Repeat.

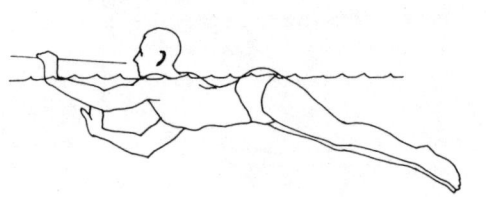

Circle Legs

Prone, holding on to pool gutter, with one hand flat on pool wall to push legs out, swimmer:

(1) Circles legs outward left.
(2) Repeat.
(3) Reverses to right.
   Repeat.

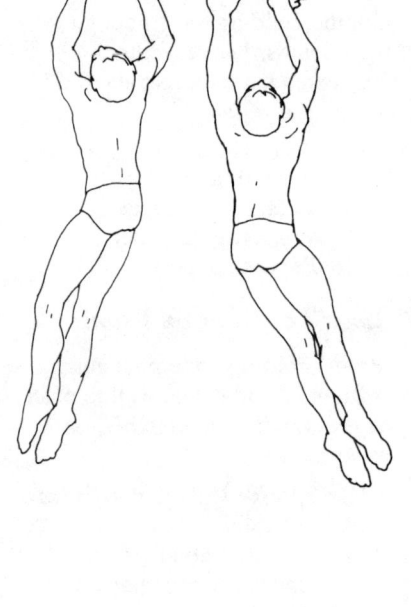

Leg Swing Outward

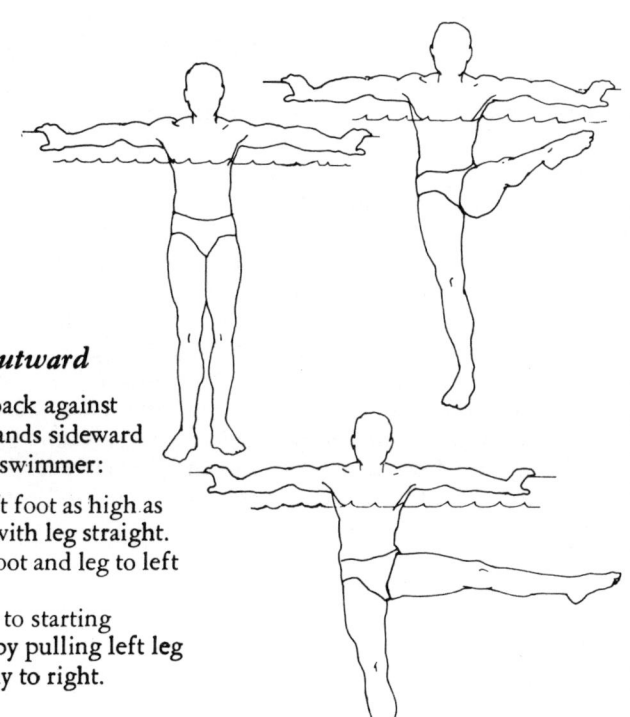

Standing with back against poolside, and hands sideward holding gutter, swimmer:

(1) Raises left foot as high as possible with leg straight.
(2) Swings foot and leg to left side.
(3) Recovers to starting position by pulling left leg vigorously to right.
Repeat.
Reverses to right leg.
Repeat.

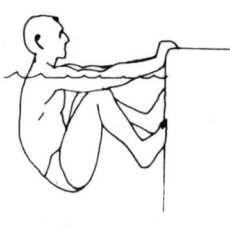

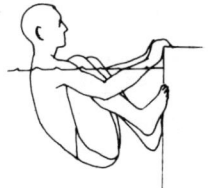

Climbing

Hands in pool gutter, facing pool side and feet flat against side and approximately 16" apart, swimmer:

(1) Walks up side by approximately six short steps.
(2) Walks down side to starting position.
Repeat.

BOBBING

An excellent conditioning activity in water is "bobbing." In "bobbing," the head and shoulders are pushed out of the water much like a cork held under water "bobs" when released. "Bobbing" is a feet-first surface dive. Some experts say that if one had only five minutes for exercise each day, it would be best to spend that time in one of four ways: 1) running, 2) trampolining, 3) rope skipping, or 4) high bobbing. During "bobbing" activities, the demands for breathing are great. "Bobbing" forces the breathing. Breathing itself is an exercise and the quick inhaling and forced exhaling requires greater effort. Maximum exertion usually demands maximum respiration. This is facilitated by regular practice of deep respirations during "bobbing". One realizes the stimulus of forced, heavy breathing after advanced "bobbing" for five minutes (approximately 100–125 times). Approximately 20 percent of Aqua Dynamics is devoted to "bobbing."

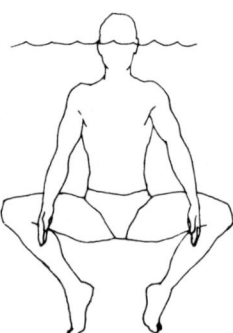

Elementary Bobbing

Standing in shallow water, swimmer:

(1) Takes a breath.
(2) Submerges in a tuck position with feet on the pool bottom in shallow water. Exhales during (2) and (3).
(3) Shoves up off the bottom and regains a standing position.
(4) Inhales with head out of water.
(5) Repeat (2), (3), (4), etc.

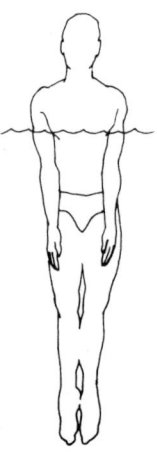

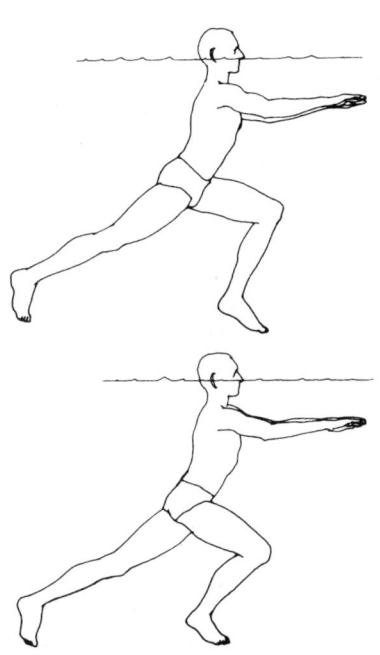

Alternate Leg Rearward Bobbing

Standing in shallow water, swimmer:

(1) Takes a breath.
(2) Submerges in shallow water with left leg in a squatting position with left foot on the pool bottom and right leg extended rearward. Exhales during (2) and (3).
(3) Shoves up off the bottom reversing the position of the legs, inhaling when the head is out of water.
(4) Submerges with right leg in a squatting position with right foot on pool bottom and left leg extended rearward. Exhales during the action.
(5) Repeat 1, 2, 3, and 4.

Alternate Leg Sideward Bobbing

Standing in waist-to-chest deep water, swimmer:

(1) Takes a breath.
(2) Submerges with left leg in a full squatting position, left foot on pool bottom and right leg extended sideward, (exhales during (2) and (3)).
(3) Shoves up off bottom reversing the position of the legs and inhaling when the head is out of water.
(4) Submerges with the right leg in a full squatting position with the right foot on pool bottom and the left leg extended sideward (exhales during the action). Repeat.

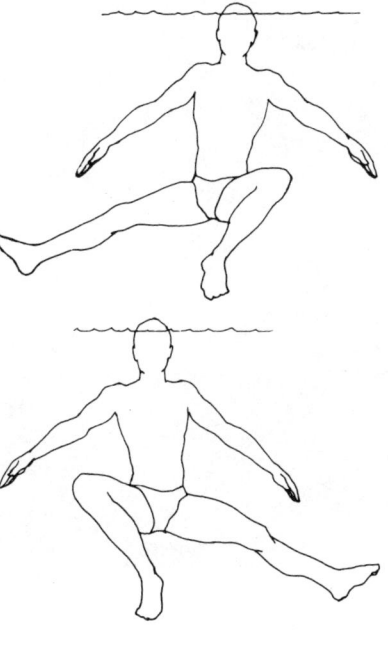

Legs Astride Bobbing

Standing in waist-to-chest deep water, swimmer:

(1) Takes a breath.
(2) Submerges with legs astride, left leg forward and right leg rearward, (exhales on (2) and (3)).
(3) Shoves off bottom, inhaling when head is out of water.
(4) Submerges with legs astride.
Repeat.

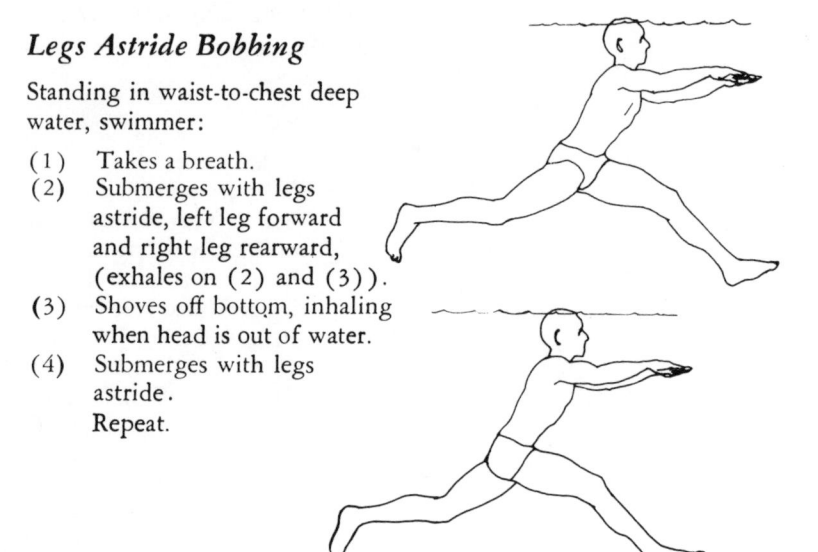

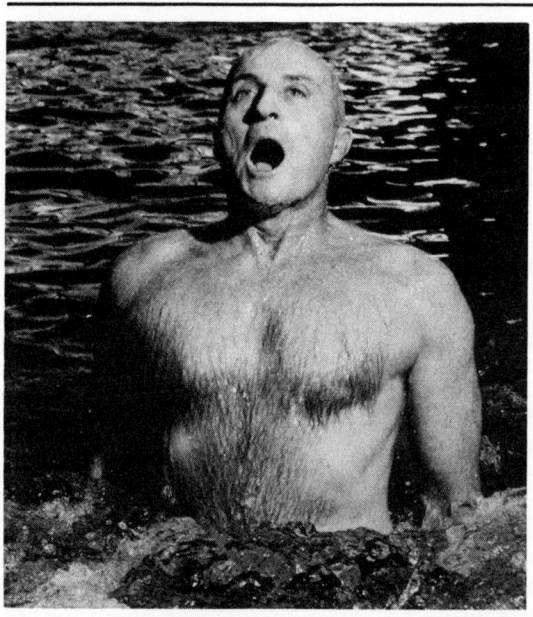

"Casey" Conrad's main water-conditioning drill is bobbing. He can bob 400 times during a one-hour workout.

Advanced Bobbing

Treading in deep water, swimmer:

(1) Assumes a vertical position with hands extended outward from the sides, just under the surface of the water, with palms turned downward. Legs are drawn in a position of readiness for a frog or scissors kick.

(2) Executes kick as hands are pulled sharply to thighs and legs. (As a result of this action, the head and shoulders rise out of the water and a deep breath is taken at the highest point reached).

(3) As the body sinks, the arms are outstretched overhead and swimmer exhales.

Repeats (1), (2), and (3).

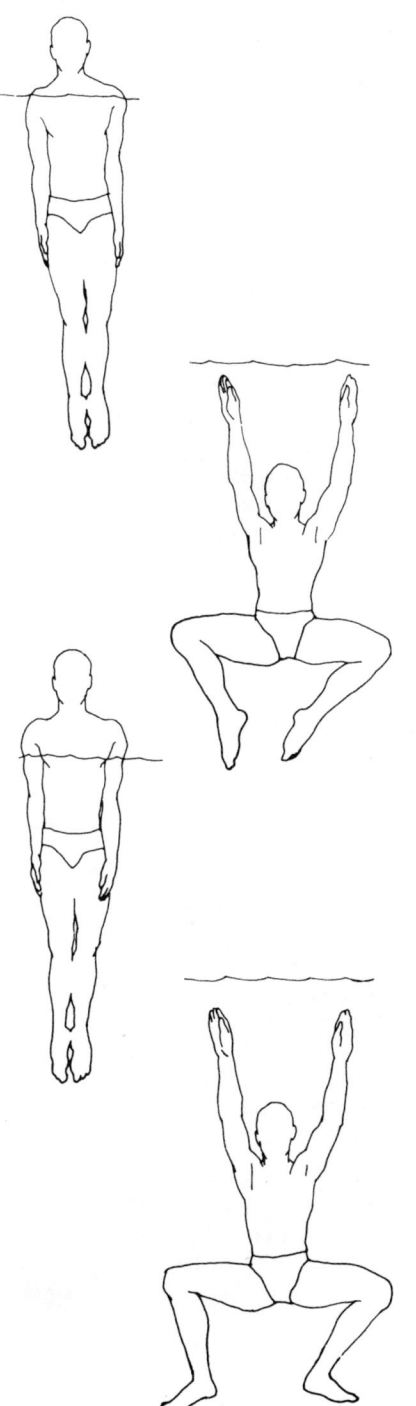

Left/Right Leg Bobbing

Standing or treading in deep water, swimmer:

(1) Takes a breath.
(2) Submerges in a tuck with right leg drawn up with left foot on pool bottom.
(3) Pushes upward off left leg thrust, exhaling during (1) and (2).
(4) Inhales with head out of water.
(5) Repeat.
Reverse to right leg.

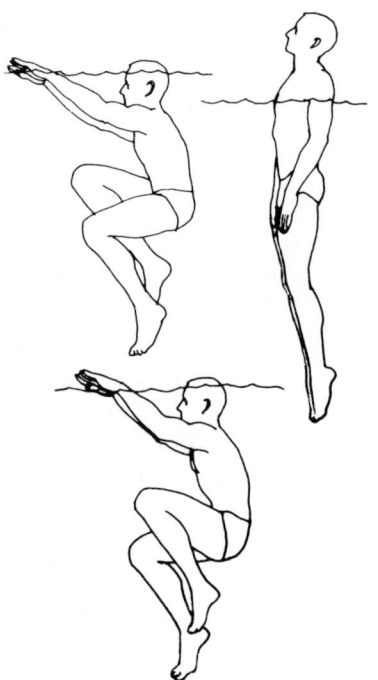

Progressive Alternate Leg Forward Bobbing

Standing, swimmer:

(1) Performs action described in Alternate Leg Rearward Bobbing (page 9), alternating legs, bobbing progressively, and moving forward the length of the pool or a specified distance.

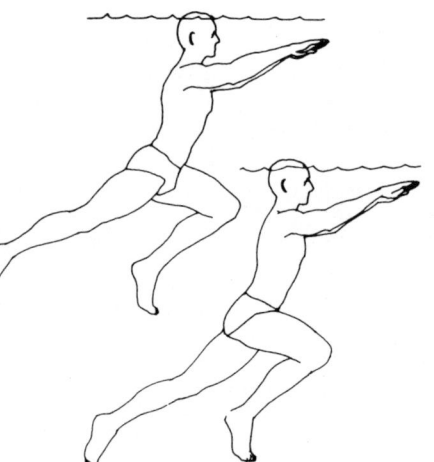

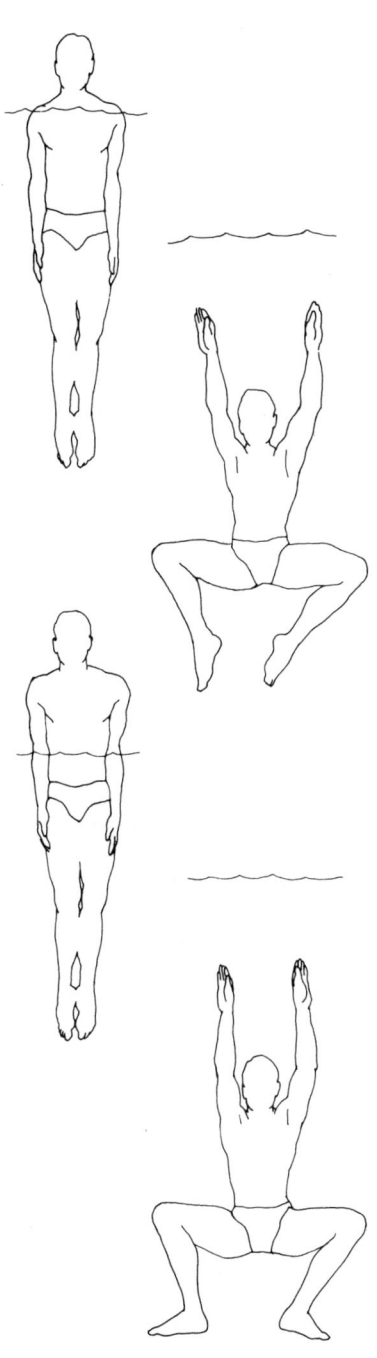

High Bobbing

In water approximately one to three feet over the swimmer's head, swimmer:

(1) Takes a vertical position, hands extended outward from the sides with palms turned downward. Legs are drawn in position for frog kick.
(2) Simultaneously pulls hands sharply to thighs with legs executing frog kick.
(3) Inhales at peak of height.
(4) Drops with thrust of arms downward with palms turned upward until feet reach bottom of the pool and tucks to a squat position. Exhales throughout this action.
(5) Jumps upward with power leg thrust at the same time pulling arms in in a breast stroke position downward, causing the head and shoulders to rise high out of water. Exhales during (4) and (5).
(6) Inhales and repeats cycles (4) and (5), etc.

Progressive "Bunny Hop" Bobbing

Standing, swimmer:

(1) Takes a breath.
(2) Submerges in a tuck or full squatting position with feet on the pool bottom.
(3) Pushes up and forward off bottom of the pool, exhaling during (2) and (3).
(4) Inhales with head out of water.
(5) Repeat, pushing forward the length of the pool or a specified distance.

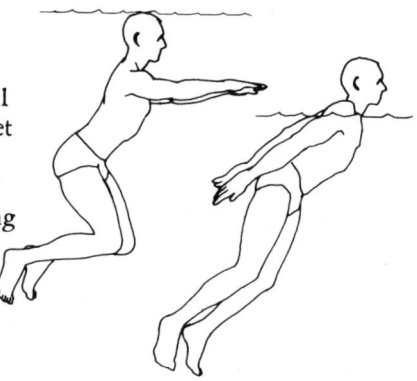

Power Bobbing

Power bobbing is similar to "high bobbing" except that at the top of the upward thrust the hands scull vigorously as the legs flutter kick. In "power bobbing" the swimmer will literally blast out of the water exposing all of the body to the hips.

Bobbing is a well-rounded workout involving leg power, arm and shoulder work, heavy forced breathing, and rhythmical vigorous action.

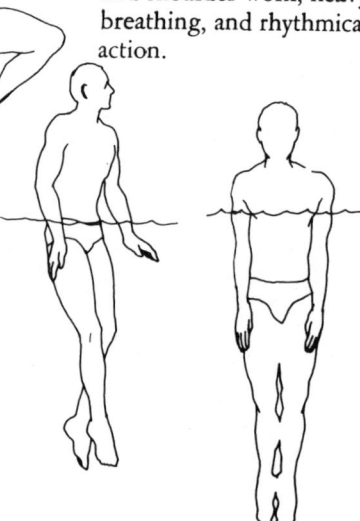

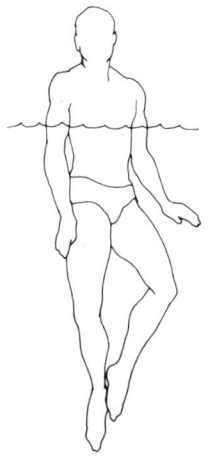

Look-Out Treading

In deep water in a perpendicular position, swimmer:

(1) Kicks vigorously at the same time thrashing the water by sculling, thereby raising the shoulders and chest high out of the water.

EXTENSIONS

Breathing

Controlled breathing is essential for the activities which follow. The swimmer should inhale through the mouth and exhale through the nose. One should be exhaling through the nose at any time the head is under water.

Sculling

"Extension" activities are largely dependent upon sculling ability. Sculling is done by arm and hand action. The use of the hands in sculling is the same basic maneuver regardless of the position of the body or the direction one wishes to go. Sculling can provide lifting power or combined lifting and propulsion power. Action usually begins by pushing down on palms, with arms sideward. Hands are flat, fingers together, and thumbs close to forefingers. With thumbs up, rotate wrists, bringing palms forward, then turn palms downward and backward. Downward pressure should be held constant on both the sideward and forward movements. Lifting power is provided as the hand is drawn to the front and side and parallel to the water surface.

Special Note: On all "extension" activities which follow, *swimmer should stay in the same place in the pool.*

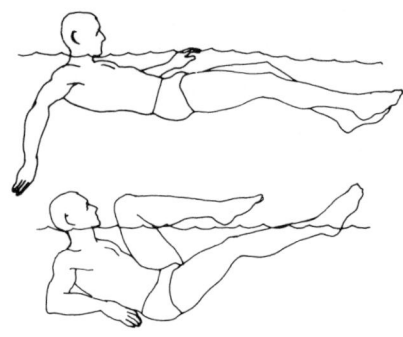

Left Knee Up, Back

Assuming a supine position, swimmer:

(1) Sculls, drawing left knee up to chest with right leg extended and toes on the right foot out of water.
(2) Sculls, straightening the left leg thus returning to the starting position. Repeat.

Right Knee Up, Back

Assuming a supine position, swimmer:

(1) Sculls, drawing right leg up to chest with left leg extended and toes on the left foot out of water.
(2) Sculls, straightening the right leg thus returning to the starting position. Repeat.

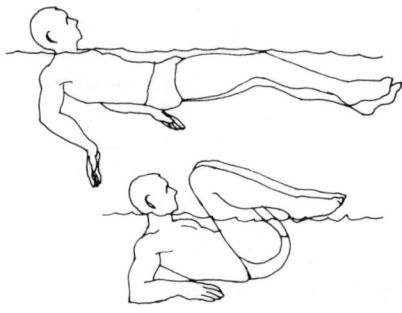

Knees Up, Back

Starting from a back-lying position, swimmer:

(1) Sculls, drawing knees up to chest.
(2) Sculls, shoving legs forward returning to a back-lying position. Repeat.

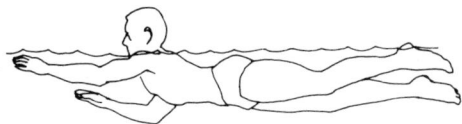

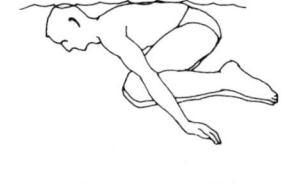

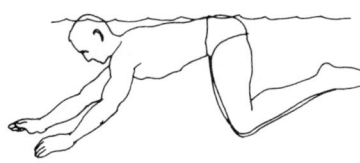

Knees Up, Front

Starting from a front-lying position, swimmer:

(1) Sculls, drawing knees up to chest.
(2) Sculls, shoving legs backward returning to the front-lying position.
Repeat.

Knees Up, Left Side

Starting from a left side stroke position, swimmer:

(1) Sculls, drawing knees up to chest.
(2) Sculls, shoving legs to the right side causing the body to be in a left side stroke position.
Repeat.

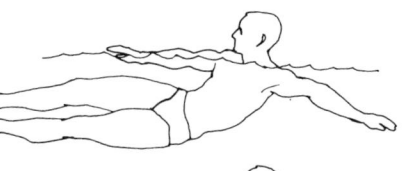

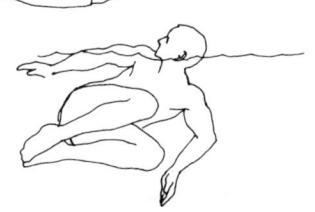

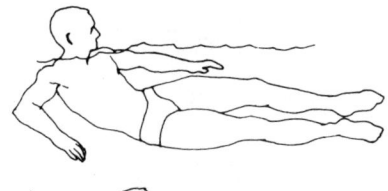

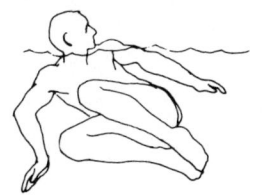

Knees Up, Right Side

Starting from a right side stroke position, swimmer:

(1) Sculls, drawing knees up to chest.
(2) Sculls, shoving legs to left side causing the body to be in a right side stroke position.
Repeat.

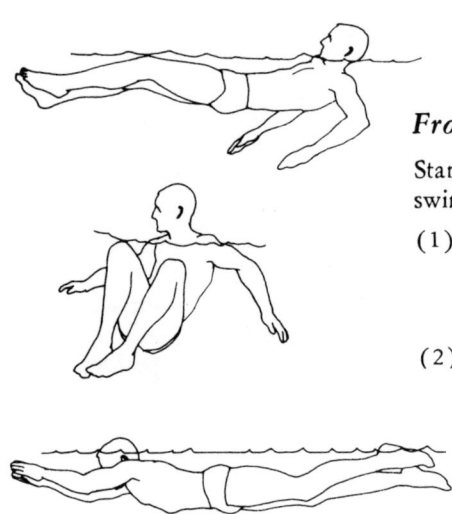

Front and Back

Starting from a vertical position, swimmer:

(1) Sculls, drawing knees up to chest, shoving legs forward coming up to a back-lying position.
(2) Sculls, drawing knees up to chest, shoving legs backward coming to a front-lying position.
Repeat.

Reverse Sides Extension

Starting from a vertical position, swimmer:

(1) Sculls, drawing knees up to chest, shoving legs to left side causing body to be in a right side stroke position.
(2) Sculls vigorously, drawing knees up to chest and reversing position; shoving legs to the right side, shifting body to a left side stroke position.
Repeat.

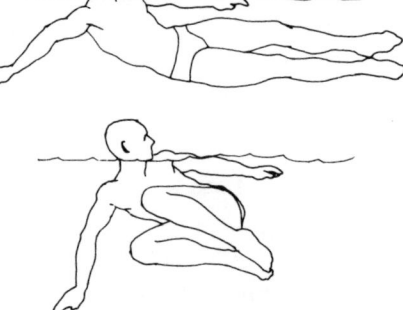

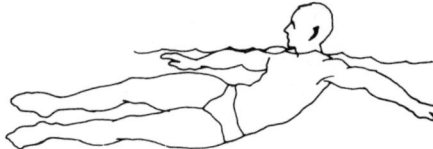

Around the Clock Extension

Starting from a vertical position, swimmer:

(1) Sculls, drawing knees up to chest, shoving legs forward to a back-lying position;
(2) Sculls vigorously, drawing knees up to chest, shoving legs to left side, causing the body to be in a right side stroke position;
(3) Sculls vigorously, drawing knees up to chest shoving the legs outward to a front-lying position; and,
(4) Sculls vigorously, drawing knees up to chest, shoving legs to right side, causing the body to be in a left side stroke position. Repeat.

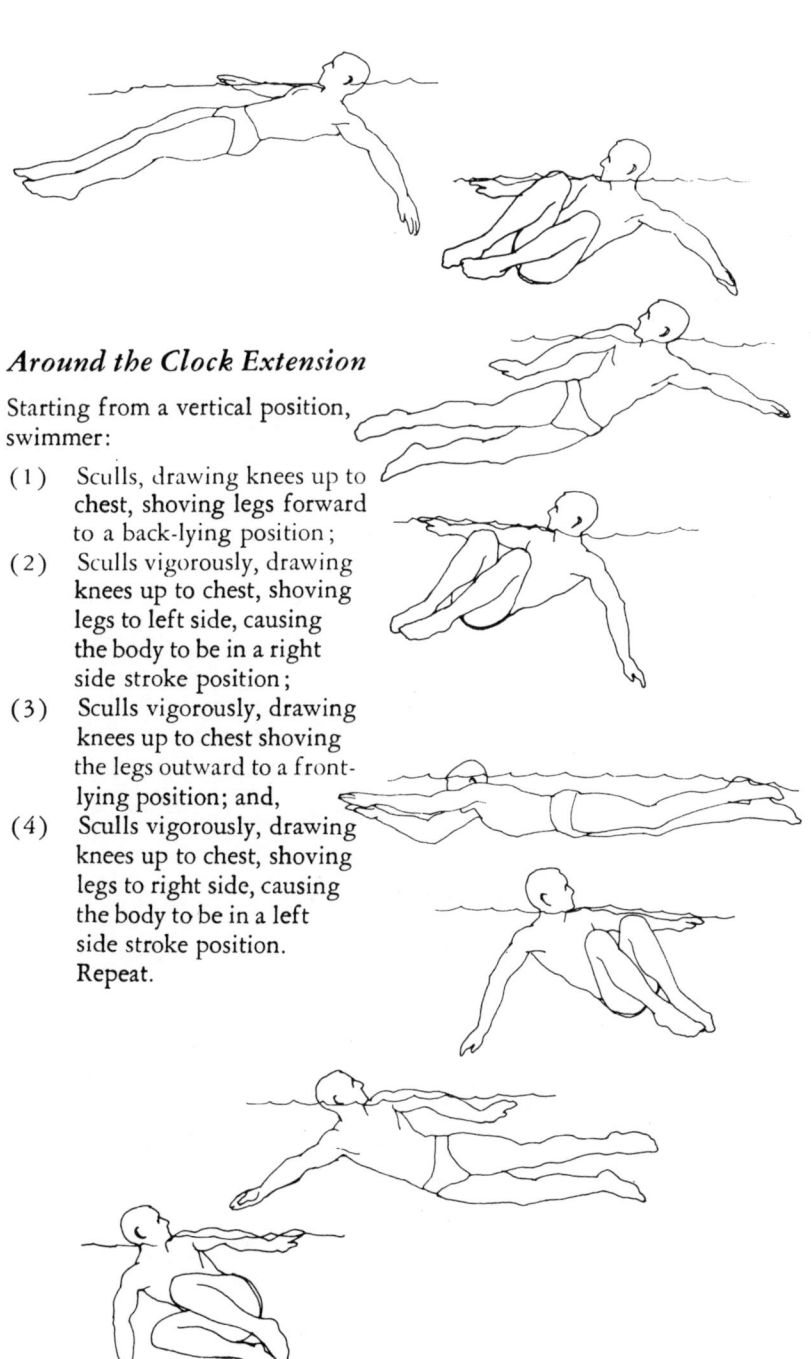

Part Three

DRESSING RICH

I remember I was relaxing on a beach on a blue-sky Sunday in August 1965, when I came across a newspaper feature story headlined "Look Out for the Men." The writer, a female fashion reporter, was the first I'd read to predict what would soon be known far and wide as the Peacock Revolution. The ground swell of a renaissance of men's interest in clothes, she said, was "as strong as the smell of fresh paint. Actually, it couldn't be more natural. Women's fashions are standing still for a while. It's women, for a change, who are in a uniform mood. Fashion is such a deep down instinct that it has to burst out somewhere. I say—look out for the men."

Soon after that, the sartorial revolution really picked up speed when women's wear designer John Weitz, following on the heels of couturiers Pierre Cardin of Paris and Hardy Amies of London, introduced a line of men's clothes. Not long afterward designer Bill Blass added a men's line to his collection, too, and then, taking a long-range look at what was happening here and abroad, commented, "We are witnessing a revolutionary awareness in men of what other men look like. Clothing has precipitated this and it will be beneficial for us all. . . . Men's awareness of what they have on their backs will intimidate the corpulent individual. Consequently, he will diet and improve his physique."

About then an elderly Englishman by the name of James Laver, a museum curator and social historian, put in an appearance in New York City to let it be known that in the pageant of history, women's fashions had just about had it for the moment. Now it was the men's turn. All this met the wholehearted approval of a reporter for the prestigious *Women's Wear Daily*. "Men," she wrote, "have sat back for too long content with the same fashions but now the revolution is on. Who can hold them back? And who

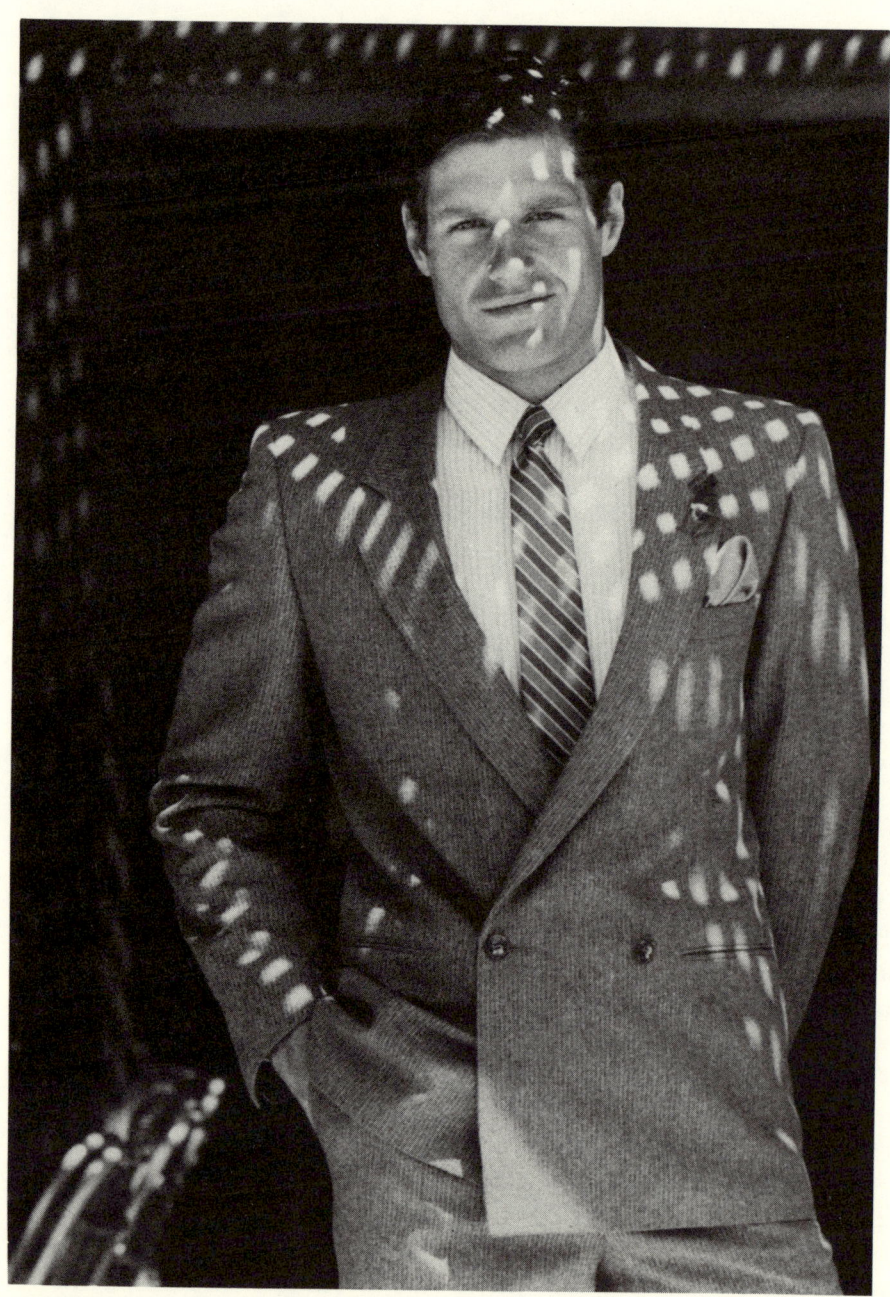
Suit by Yves Saint Laurent. PHOTO COURTESY OF J. P. STEVENS & CO., INC.

would want to hold those handsome cats back from looking even better?"

Before long Joe Namath was posing for the press in a $5,000 double-breasted mink overcoat, and in 1968 the Best-Dressed Men's list was compiled for the first time with this accompanying explanation: "Men's clothes are now too important a part of the fashionable scene to ignore the creative leadership of certain men as symbols of the best in contemporary masculine dress." Translation: *Men's fashions had become big business.* Whereas a man's clothes used to be "out" when they wore out, they were now subject to the calculated whims of fashion pundits.

The rest is history. The Peacock Revolution catapulted some men out of their natural-shoulder suits, button-down shirts, and skinny ties into Nehru jackets, turtleneck sweaters, and love beads and, in the process, some people maintain, set men's fashions back twenty years. Anyway, by 1971 *GQ (Gentlemen's Quarterly)* magazine was announcing on its cover, "The Costume Party Is Over!" The editors heralded the return of the gentleman; the excesses of the fashion revolution were a thing of the past. Hallelujah!

So where are we now? A whole lot more receptive to new ideas in fashion than we've ever been before and far more relaxed about what we put on our backs. That's a legacy of the Peacock Revolution we can all be thankful for. Clothing, after all, should be used to make our lives easier.

Elegance today is both comfortable and spontaneous-looking and, I'm sorry to say, a lot more expensive to achieve. Today, when you pay more to buy a suit off the rack than it cost to order one custom-made on London's Savile Row only ten years ago, it behooves a man to shop with considerable savvy and to take very special care of what he buys, to know something about colors and patterns and how to mix them.

There are two pieces of fashion advice I think every mature man should follow: One, never dress purposely young and trendy; two, dress for your way of life.

Dressing young and trendy is a sure way to call attention to the fact you're past the first flush of youth. It's a simple matter of practicality when buying clothes to stay true to your life-style while paying close attention to quality and price. I often think that Emily Post, the longtime arbiter of etiquette, said it all when she commented in reference to a man's business wear, "Whatever the fashion of the moment, if a man's suit fits him well, is appropriate to whatever he may be doing, and is not overly conspicuous in style or color, he may rest assured that he will be labeled well-dressed in any community."

Men communicate with one another through their clothes. The clothes you wear and how you choose to wear them send out messages about your social stratum, sensibility, mobility, and cash or credit position. With that firmly in mind, let's now get down to the nitty-gritty:

1. Dress stylishly conservative, choose clothing that's simply cut, and you can't go wrong. Men's clothes are becoming simpler, more relaxed, less dressy.

2. Buy the best-quality fabrics. They last longer and clean better.

3. Comfort means clothes that fit easily and move with your body.

4. Never dress "young." Aim, instead, to look well cared for, vital—eternally forty.

5. Periodically weed out your wardrobe, and get rid of clutter. If you have things you haven't worn in a long time, chances are that you've already mentally chucked them out. Now go ahead and do it physically.

Under the title "First Class Male," *W*, the semimonthly fashion newspaper published by Fairchild Publications, listed what it called "The no nos." Here are the ones having to do with fashion:

Leisure or pleasure suits	Undershirts
White patent leather shoes	Too-short pants
Anything initialed, except shirts, discreetly	Flashy colors, prints and plaids
Chunky buckled belts and shoes	Chest-baring shirts
	Nautical motifs
Big chains and medallions	Emblemed blazers
Jumpsuits	Sandals with socks
Fake leather trim	Colored evening shirts
Robes at the beach or pool	Patched blue jeans and patched jackets that aren't old
Bikinis	
Belts that don't buckle	
Pants tucked in boots	Car Coats
Handbags	

Elsewhere the editors illustrated some fashions that won approval. Here are some: a gold tie bar from Cartier; a reversible brown to black calf belt; cotton denim blue jeans; a black mohair-and-wool dinner suit; sueded pigskin gloves with cashmere lining; a classic button-down blue cotton oxford shirt from Brooks Brothers; a double-breasted camel's hair coat; brown leather loafers from Gucci; a set of three linen handkerchiefs; a classic trench coat with button-out melton lining; charcoal gray flannel pants; a pigskin wallet; a classic single-breasted navy wool blazer; and a gray cashmere V-neck pullover.

Of course, you don't have to agree with everything on either list. I like white patent leather shoes, for example. But lists like these do give you some indication of what's happening in those pockets of the fashion world where the image makers get together.

SUITS

What is the bare minimum a man who wants to look his best at all times can get by with? An Italian designer from Milan says, "An elegant man needs to have forty suits of all types." Digest that, and then move on fast for other opinions.

According to designer Bill Blass, three suits would cover all neces-

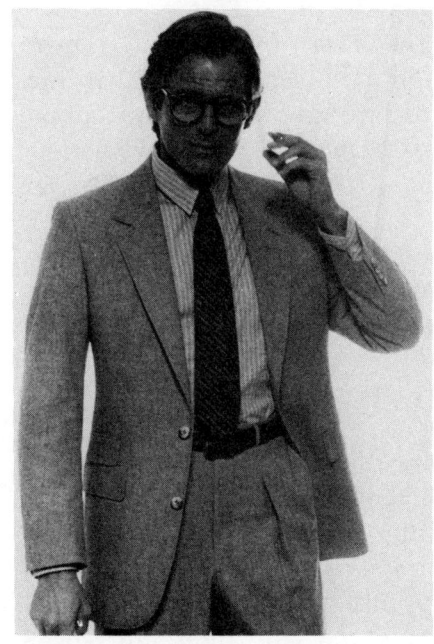

SUIT BY BILL BLASS.

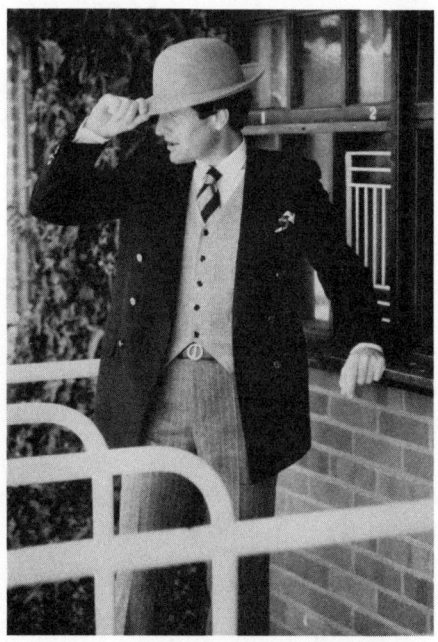

SUIT BY ALFRED DUNHILL OF LONDON.

sities in a man's life: a gray flannel ("A man's never without a gray flannel suit"), a navy serge, and a chalk stripe.

British designer Hardy Amies, whose men's clothes sell both here and abroad and who was one of the first "name" designers to enter the menswear field, elaborates:

"Put as much money as you can muster into a blazer suit. By that I mean a blazer with brass buttons and a pair of trousers in the same cloth—all lightweight, largely wool, in navy blue or, better still, what I call a midnight blue. You could even wear this as a dinner suit, with a white shirt, a black satin tie, and black leather moccasins. With a white shirt and a knitted blue tie you could wear your blazer suit to any cocktail party at any embassy anywhere in the world. Buy a pair of gray flannel trousers, and it's another outfit. Buy three pairs of khaki chinos (three pairs because that way you can always have a clean pair), and a couple of cashmere sweaters with round necks—one long-sleeved and one sleeveless. Then one sports jacket in a sort of deep oatmeal shade you can wear with your gray flannel and your chinos, and if you've kept a good figure and have a nice tanned face, you're going to look great—absolutely great!"

What to Look for When Buying a Suit

Fabric. Finished suitings, and the yarns from which they're made, fall into two classes: worsted and woolen. Serge, gabardine, and sharkskin are examples of worsted suitings; tweed is an example of woolen suitings. Flannel and covert may be either woolen or worsted, proving only that you can't always depend on the name of the cloth to tell you which it is.

Worsted yarns are generally close-woven, hard-finished, supple, and smooth. Crumple a piece of worsted, and it will spring back *sans* wrinkles. Woolen yarns are coarser, have a softer finish, and are usually more loosely twisted than worsteds. While they generally don't keep their shape or press as well as worsted, woolens don't wrinkle all that readily.

Since fabric accounts for about one-third of the cost of a suit's manufacture, doesn't it make sense that you should know something about it? Ideally it should be supple to the touch. "The closer to wood the fabric feels, the cheaper it is," says Norman Block, president of the world-renowned Dunhill Tailors.

The following table of spring-summer and fall-winter suit fabrics

Spring-Summer Fabrics

	Cleans	Holds Shape	Wrinkles
Cord	Dry clean	Fairly well	Moderately
Covert	Wash and Dry	Fairly well	Moderately
Gabardine	Dry clean	Well	Slightly
Hopsack	Dry clean	Fairly well	Readily
Knit	Dry clean	Extraordinarily well	Crease-resistant
Linen	Wash and Dry or Dry clean	Briefly	Readily
Oxford cloth	Wash and Dry	Fairly well	Readily
Polyester and Acrylic fibers	Wash and Dry	Well	Moderately
Polyester, Mohair, and Worsted	Dry clean	Very well	Moderately
Polyester and Rayon	Wash and Dry	Well	Moderately
Polyester and Wool	Dry clean	Well	Good wrinkle resistance
Polyester and Worsted	Dry clean	Fairly well	Good wrinkle resistance
Poplin	Wash and Dry	Fairly well	Moderately
Seersucker: All cotton	Wash and Dry	Fairly well	Moderately
Seersucker: Polyester and Cotton	Wash and Dry	Well	Moderately
Silk	Dry clean	Fairly well	Moderately
Stretch Poplin	Dry clean	Fairly well	Good wrinkle resistance
Velvet	Dry clean	Fairly well	Good wrinkle resistance
Velveteen	Dry clean	Fairly well	Good wrinkle resistance

	Cleans	Holds Shape	Wrinkles
Worsted:			
Tropical	Dry clean	Extremely well	Good wrinkle resistance
Worsted and Mohair	Dry clean	Extremely well	Good wrinkle resistance

Fall-Winter Fabrics

	Cleans	Holds Shape	Wrinkles
Cashmere and Wool	Dry clean	Briefly	Moderately
Cavalry Twill	Dry clean	Very well	Good wrinkle resistance
Cheviot	Dry clean	Fairly well	Readily
Corduroy	Wash and Dry or Dry clean	Fairly well	Good wrinkle resistance
Flannel	Dry clean	Fairly well	Moderately
Hopsack	Dry clean	Fairly well	Moderately
Serge	Dry clean	Very well	Good wrinkle resistance
Sharkskin	Dry clean	Well	Slightly
Tweed	Dry clean	Briefly	Readily
Whipcord	Dry clean	Very well	Slightly
Wool and Acrylic blend	Dry clean	Fairly well	Readily

will give you some clue as to their durability and performance.

Lining should be smoothly fitted and fine-stitched by hand with matching silk thread. A cheap rayon lining often shrinks and puckers during dry cleaning. The best lining material is a synthetic fabric from Germany known by the brand name Bemberg; it's silky smooth and extraordinarily durable.

A full lining, however, is not necessarily a sign of a fine suit. Today many expensive suits have only a half or three-quarter lining. In any case, whatever seams you see should be neatly finished off.

Trousers of a rough-textured fabric should also have a lining for comfortable wear. A suit made of a soft fabric—cashmere or camel's hair, for example—should also be lined to minimize sagging.

Look, too, for still another form of lining at the base of the armhole: the triangular flap (sweat shield) that's found in any really well-made suit.

Sleeves, properly cut, should taper to the cuff with the top of the sleeve looking smooth and round, with nary a wrinkle. Of course, one-quarter inch of shirt cuff should show at the wrist.

Shoulders. Fabric should be smooth at the shoulders. There should be a firm, unbroken shoulderline from the neck to the shoulder point. Watch out for a horizontal ripple below the base of the neck—a warning that material should be cut away across the top of the shoulder. Stand tall, and note if there are tension lines tugging between the shoulder blades. If there are, the back is too tight and should be let out. There should be a straight line with no wrinkles from the shoulder to the lower edge of the coat, back and front.

The acid test when trying on a new jacket: Raise both arms

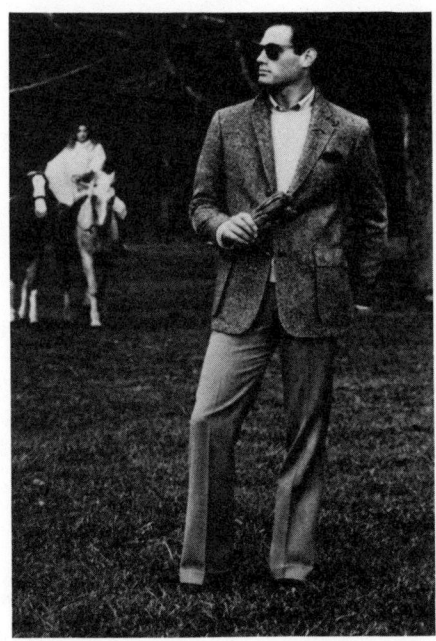

SUIT BY CRICKETEER, A DIVISION OF PHILLIPS VAN HEUSEN CORP.

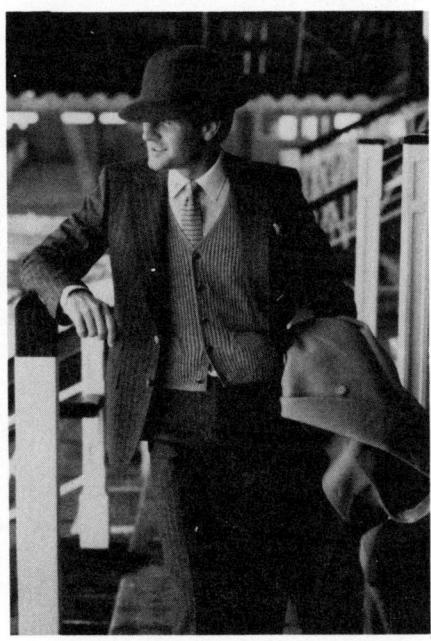

SUIT BY ALFRED DUNHILL OF LONDON.

over your head, and then bring them down, slowly, to your sides. The jacket should settle comfortably on your shoulders without the fabric's bunching around the collar, or under the arms.

Armholes should be cut high rather than low. Cut too low, and the sleeve will bind when you raise your arm.

Collar fit should be low and close to the back and sides of the neck, allowing about five-eighths of an inch of shirt collar showing in the back over the suit collar.

Waist. Button the coat, and if horizontal creases show up in the small of the back or you see X-shaped lines radiating out from the top button, the waist is too tight.

Trousers. How much flare your trousers have depends pretty much on your height and build. The tall, thin man usually looks best with flare and cuffs to break up an excessively long-legged look; the portly man looks best in tapered trousers without cuffs. But plain or cuffed, trousers should hang straight to the shoe without a break in front. A deep break makes trousers look too long. On the other hand, your socks should never be visible unless you're seated; too short trousers give a man that golly-gee Li'l Abner look. In the back the trousers should slant to hang one-quarter inch over the back of the shoe.

Advice from some quarters would have you reserve trouser cuffs for sport and country wear. I consider that nonsense. If you feel comfortable in cuffed trousers, wear them whenever you wish.

As for the waistband, determine if it has an inner or double curtain lining. That's the sole guarantee you have against the unsightly rollover that can show up when you've worn the trousers a couple of times.

Vest fit should be smooth and close—a kind of second skin. Traditionally, the last button is always left undone.

Pockets should lie flat and smooth. Opt for one or two inside breast pockets, one to carry your pocket wallet for safety's sake. It should go without saying that your wallet should be lean and flat so as not to interfere with the line of your jacket.

Pattern. Check the matching of the material. The pattern of the material should match at the seams. This is especially important with plaids, stripes, and fabrics with designs.

The above are guidelines, not hard 'n' fast rules. Much depends on a man's proportions, and the very best test for what looks best on you is to check it out yourself before a three-way mirror.

Fashion Tips

FOR THE SHORT MAN

Wear	*Avoid*
Solid-color suits for an illusion of more height	Bold plaids
Vertical patterned designs	Hip-hugger-style trousers
Uncuffed trousers	Flared trousers
A longer lapel on your jacket	Pockets with flaps

FOR THE TALL, THIN MAN

Wear	*Avoid*
Suit shoulders as squared as fashion permits	An extremely shaped suit
Double-breasted jackets and flapped pockets	Fabrics that cling
Low-rise, hip-hugger-style trousers	Very dark colors
Wider, lower-cut lapels	
Checks, overplaid, and glenurquhart plaids	

FOR THE FAT MAN

Wear	*Avoid*
Suit jacket shoulders slightly padded to avoid any suggestion of tightness	Necessarily accepting the dictum that you look best in a single-breasted suit. A lot depends on your proportions. For some overweight men, a double-breasted style tends to flatten a bulging abdomen
Jacket and trousers only slightly tapered	Center vents
Smooth suiting fabrics (gabardines, sharkskins, etc.) in medium and dark colors	Low-rise, hip-hugger-style trousers
Small, quiet patterns	Tweeds and bulk fabrics
Side vents	Cuffed trousers and pocket flaps

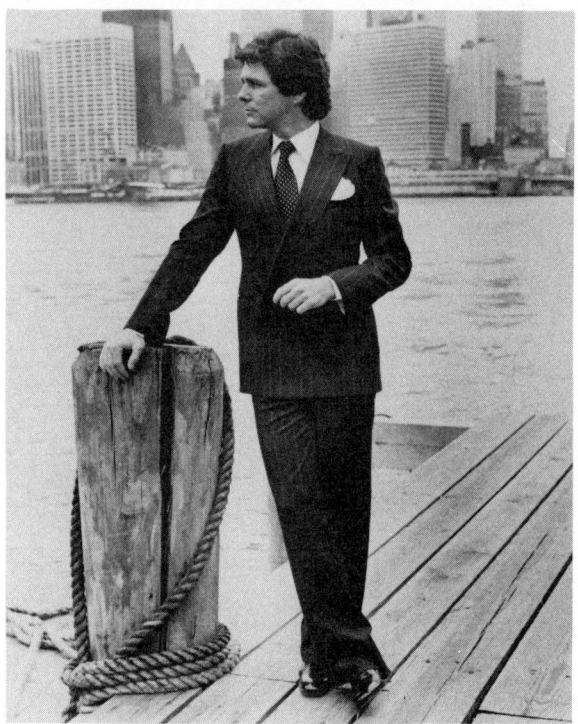
SUIT BY DIMITRI OF ITALY, INC.

Tips on Caring for Your Suits

1. Suits should be dry-cleaned on an average of once every eight wearings and pressed twice as often. Why more pressing? Well, if it's done with a professional steam iron, the steam forced through the fabric has the effect of a semicleaning.

2. As soon as a suit comes back from the cleaner's, transfer it to a wishbone-shaped wooden hanger.

3. Leather buttons on a sports jacket? Ask your cleaner to cover them with foil before cleaning, or there's a better than fair chance that the cleaning process will strip them of color.

4. It's a good idea to brush a suit after wearing it. It will help preserve the fabric's nap. For a tweed, use a long-bristled brush; for smooth-finish fabrics, simply wrap some adhesive tape around your hand—sticky side out—and pat all over the suit.

How to Take Your Own Measurements

There are some dandy slacks that can be ordered by mail. But how do you take your own waist and inseam measurements accurately? With a tape measure held straight and snug, but not taut.

Waist Size. Place the tape measure around your waist over the shirt (not slacks) at the height you usually wear your slacks. Bear in mind that because jeans can come in low-rise, medium-rise, or regular-rise styles, you must check description and illustration most carefully so you measure at the correct point on your body. Keep one finger between tape and body. The number of inches is your waist size.

Inseam Length. Lay a pair of well-fitting slacks flat with crease at back and front. Fold one leg back, and measure from the crotch, along inseam, to length preferred. The number of inches is your inseam length.

SHIRTS AND TIES

What with so many men exercising regularly these days, it's wise to check out neck and sleeve size now and then. A more muscular back, for instance, affects sleeve length. So using the trusty tape measure again, here's how it goes.

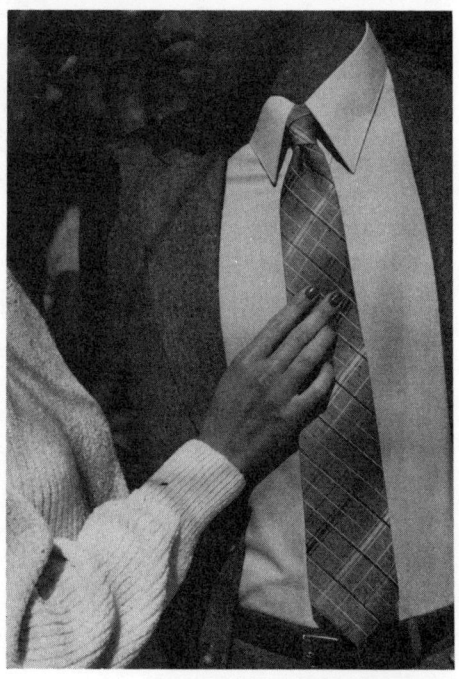

A Wembley tie.

158   THE MATURE MAN'S GUIDE TO STYLE

Sleeve Length. Bend elbow, measure from center of neck (back side) to elbow and up wrist. The number of inches equals your size.

Neck Size. On a shirt that fits you well, lay the collar flat, and measure it from center of collar button to far end of collar buttonhole. The number of inches is your neck size.

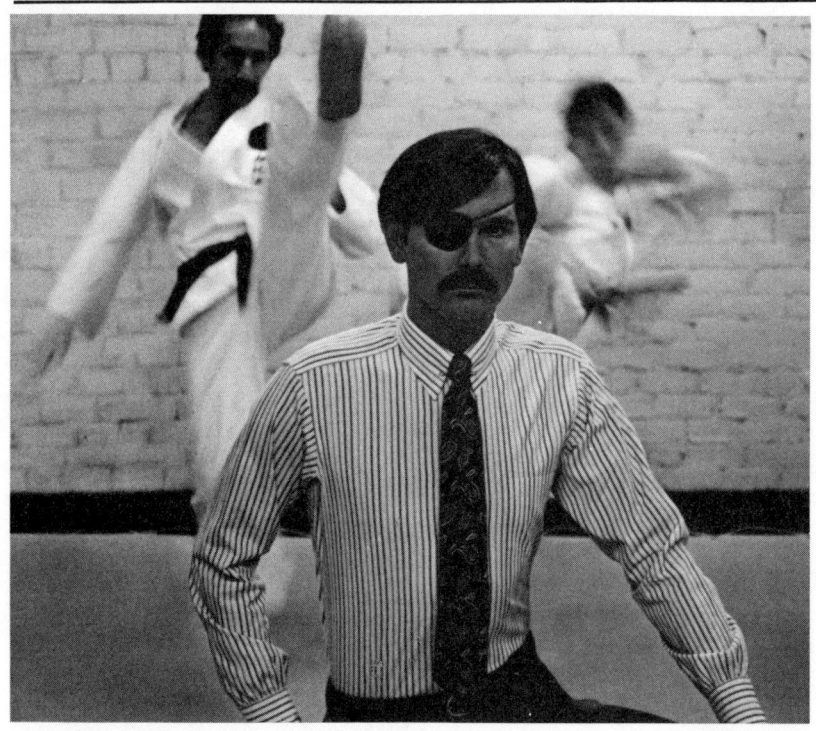

SHIRT BY C. F. HATHAWAY.

Shirt Talk

There's something comfortable and reassuring about being able to talk knowledgeably about shirts to a shirt salesman, to know, for instance, what "permanent press" really means. So here's a fast and easy course in Shirt Talk.

Permanent press also goes under the name of durable press, and under either name it simply means that the shirt fabric has been chemically treated and heat-cured. Result: permanent shape-retaining and wrinkle-shedding properties.

Wash-and-wear means that the shirting fabric has been heat-treated and resin-coated so that it can be run through the wash and spin cycles of an automatic washer, dried in an automatic dryer, and worn again with little or no pressing.

Sanforized is the registered brand name of a process for shrink resistance. It means that such a shirt will shrink no more than a fraction of 1 percent.

Barrel cuff is the name given to the basic button-fastened cuff. The name applies no matter how many buttons and buttonholes.

French cuff is twice the length of the barrel cuff and is worn folded back with the two halves held together with cuff links.

Convertible cuff has a buttonhole on both ends plus a small button so that you have a choice of wearing it buttoned or with cuff links.

Point length refers to the distance between the top edge of the collar to the tip of the collar tips.

Spread refers to the distance between the tips of the two collar tips.

Slope refers to the height of the collar on the neck. All collar styles are usually available in a choice of regular, high, or low slope.

Choosing Your Most Flattering Collar Style

The collar is the key to a shirt's style; it's the most noticeable part of your shirt. And the shape of your face is the determining factor in choosing a collar style. Which is yours—broad, long and narrow, oval? Well, according to *Esquire* magazine of July 1979 there's one foolproof way to decide:

Lay a ruler flat on your shaving mirror, and put your nose against the glass. Mark with your fingers the distance between your cheekbones. If it's more than five inches, yours is a broad face. If it's around four inches, it's narrow, and it looks still narrower if you measure more than eight inches from brow to chin. Somewhere in between, you're probably the basic oval.

The broad face almost always has a short neck. Long collars—three inches or more, no less than two and seven-eighth inches—with moderate spreads are the answer. The popular button-down collar with long points, for example, looks extremely attractive. So do shirts with color-contrasting collars. Rounded pin collars, on the other hand, are to be avoided since they give a tight look around the neck, as are very wide bow ties.

The long, narrow face looks especially good in a spread collar. Collars should be two and seven-eighth inches long, and they can be shortened with a collar pin or with a button-down style. Avoid wide, short collars and very wide bow ties (they narrow a narrow face just as they blow up a broad face).

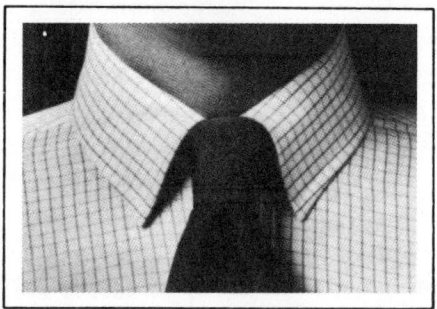

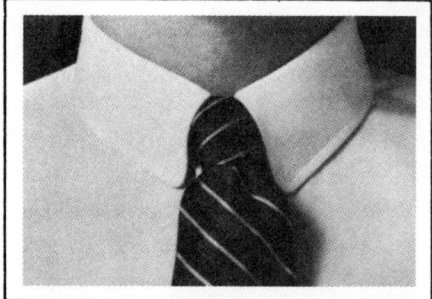
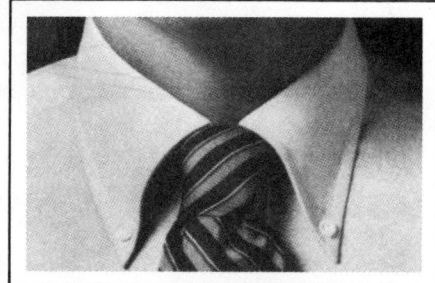

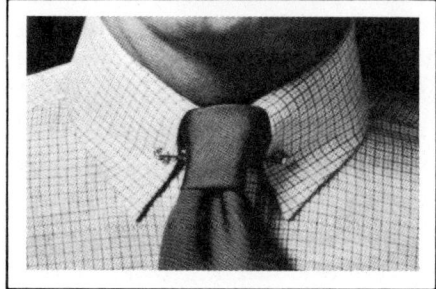
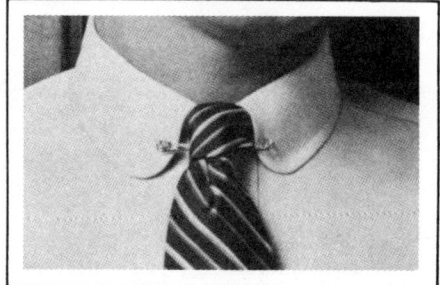

PHOTOS COURTESY OF C. F. HATHAWAY.

The oval face has only one style to avoid: the rounded collar. It produces a monotonous, too-many-smooth-curves look. Best bets: collars two and a half inches or so in length—even longer.

A Question of Color

Years ago a businessman intent on moving up the corporate ladder had a wardrobe of white shirts. But by 1973, when I was writing a magazine article on men's fashions, the blue-chip corporations were taking a more liberated attitude toward seeing their men in more colorful garb. I recall an executive at the Ford Motor Company in Dearborn telling me, "Colored and striped shirts are the major change you see at Ford. And that's a welcome change from white and blue."

However, in 1979 Stanley Hyman, president of Identity Research Institute, an organization concerned with "the research and application of behavioral sciences," was telling an audience of 150 men that suits with vests look authoritative and symbolize sincerity and that shirts should be white ("nothing has more integrity"). But speaking to the same audience that day, another lecturer contended that "white drains color from your face; colored shirts bring out the color of your suit."

Personally I like colored shirts. White is hard to wear, particularly for the man with gray or white hair unless he has a ruddy or tanned complexion. A shirt of ivory or bone color is close to white but much more flattering for most men.

When choosing a colored shirt, bear this in mind: Its purpose is to flatter your skin tone, not to overpower it.

Tips on Caring for Your Shirts

1. Wear a shirt once, and put it aside for laundering. Wear it twice without laundering, and body oils and dirt will abbreviate its life span.

2. When putting on your tie, don't leave the shirt collar up, Instead, fold it down, and slip the tie under it to keep the collar neat.

3. Before putting a wet shirt on a hanger to dry, place a dry towel around the hanger first. It takes all of six seconds but helps retain collar shape and avoids rust marks from the hanger.

4. Does anybody want a shirt starched anymore? I think not. A well-made shirt of a good fabric certainly doesn't require it, and more to the point, constant starching shortens the life span of the shirt.

5. Make it a habit before tossing a shirt into the hamper to remove collar stays; if you send a shirt to the laundry with the stays intact, they'll melt into the fabric during pressing.

6. Naturally you apply your deodorant before dressing, but be sure to let it dry before you put your shirt on. Some deodorants while still damp can stain shirting fabrics.

7. White buttons can come back from the laundry yellow-tinged from the ironing. Rubbing with a clean ink eraser has been known to restore their pearly-looking quality.

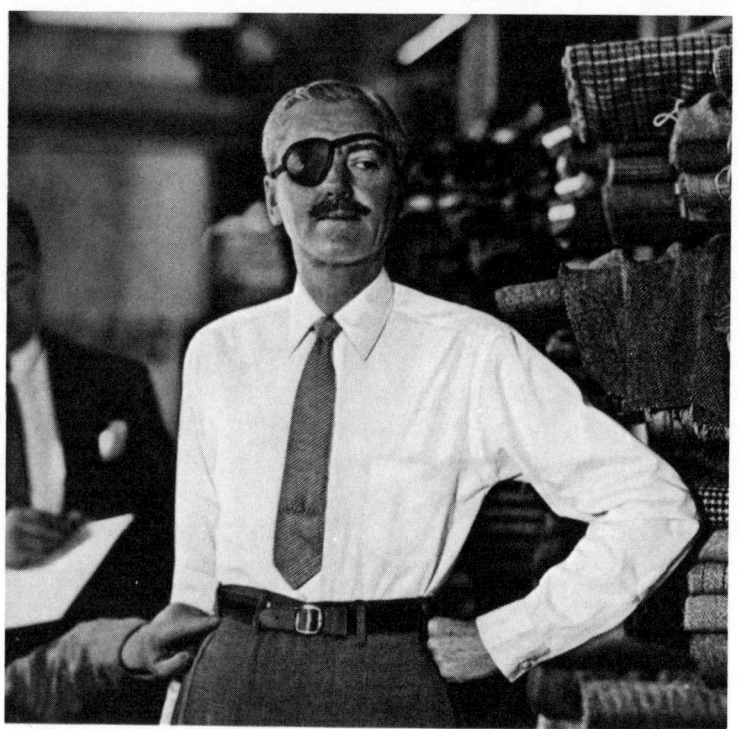

Hathaway's first "eyepatch" ad, circa 1951.

Tie Talk

Proportion's the key factor: narrower ties for shorter collars, larger knots for wider spreads.

A good interlining allows a tie to knot easily and stay wrinkle-free and gives it a luxurious feel; muslin is the best interlining.

Linen ties look smart, but linen is a fragile fabric. It's better to settle for an imitation or linen blend.

Speaking to *The New York Times* about men's current receptiveness to new fashion ideas, designer Geoffrey Beene said that by the 1980s many men may even be willing to give up their ties "if we designers can think of something feasible to replace them." Perhaps, but I doubt it because no other item of apparel in a man's wardrobe gives him as much opportunity to express his personality. Last year Americans spent some $800 million on ties.

Syndicated columnist John Molloy, author of the best-selling book *Dress for Success*, calls the tie "the heraldic shield of the 20th century. It tells who you are and where you're going." He states that in about 95 percent of the corporations in America the tie is a symbol not just that you have power but that you even have the potential of power. Molloy claims that ties of a darker color are more authoritative, as are smaller patterns. He recommends, "If you're going to an important meeting, wear a small-patterned maroon tie."

Designer John Weitz says the tie is "a man's personal battle flag. It's the equivalent of the Western bandanna or the yachtsman's private flag. It's the only chance in the day for a man to be frivolous. It also gives him his only artistic opportunity; there's not much you can do with putting on a shirt or trousers, but you have to tie a tie."

Dr. Ernest Dichter, a motivational psychologist, says "a tie exposes and covers up at the same time. What it exposes is the personality of the wearer. What it covers is the shirtfront." A tie is also, he claims, a symbol of virility. Tieless men, he says, are very unsure of their sexuality.

How to Tie One On

We all know the steps, but many of us do them rather haphazardly so that the end result is a lot less refined-looking than it should be. A little thoughtful practice might be in order.

The four-in-hand—the knot most frequently seen—is the name derived indirectly from the driver of the coach drawn by four horses, in two teams in tandem, with the lines of all four held in one hand. The driver wore a slipknot tie, which became known as the four-in-hand. Here's how it's tied.

1. Cross the long end over the short end.
2. Bring long end under short end.
3. Bring long end around short end.
4. Bring long end through center at top.
5. Pull long end through loop and form center crease.
6. Slide completed knot into place.

The Windsor has been in hiding since the advent of the wide tie in the late sixties. After all, the wide tie made a very wide knot, and who needed to tie a wide, triangular Windsor knot? Well, the narrow tie has made a comeback, as has the Windsor knot, so called because the late Duke of Windsor, the most potent fashion figure of this century, wore large-knot ties in the 1930s. By the way, wide ties worn with the Windsor knot help balance a tall, thin man's vertical lines. And now here's a refresher course on how to tie one on.

1. Cross the long end over the short end.
2. Loop the long end under and over the short end and then under again.
3. Bring the long end up over the neckband and down toward the other side.
4. Wrap the long end around the front of the knot; then loop it under the neckband and down through the loop.
5. Slide the completed knot in place.

The half Windsor is, as its name implies, only half as bulky as the Windsor. Still, it's recommended only for wide ties with lightweight fabrics that aren't heavily lined.

1. Start with the wide end on your right, hanging about a foot below the narrow end.
2. Cross the wide end over the narrow; then turn it back underneath.
3. Bring it up over the neckband and down through the opposite side.
4. Pass it around the front, from left to right.
5. Take it up underneath through the neckband.
6. Finally, pass it down through the knot in front. Tighten it carefully—not too tight—and draw it up to the collar.

The Bow Tie

Bows come in a variety of widths, but if it's a hand-tied bow rather than a pretied bow, you tie them all the same way. Personally I find a bow tie a spirit lifter, and furthermore, it has a kind of rejuvenating effect on a man's face.

1. Start with both ends of the tie hanging evenly.
2. Slide the left end down until it hangs approximately 1½ inches below the right end.
3. Cross the long end over the short, and pass it underneath the loop that you've just made.
4. Double up the short end, and place it across the collar points, centered about where the finished knot will be.
5. Hold it there with the thumb and forefinger of the left hand, and drop the low end down over the front.
6. Place the right forefinger, pointing up, on the bottom

half of the hanging part. Now pass it up underneath the loop formed by the short end.

7. The result is another loop, which you poke through the knot behind the front loop.

8. Tug, twist, even up until both ends are as wide as the spread of your eyes.

HOW TO COORDINATE COLORS AND PATTERNS

A blue suit looks good on every man, probably the reason why it's a staple in most men's wardrobes. It is especially flattering for men with gray or white hair. The only color shirts to avoid when wearing a blue suit are tan and green. When it comes to selecting a tie for a blue suit, red, maroon, blue, light gray, gold, and ivory should be at the top of your color list; a brown or tan tie isn't to be considered.

A brown suit looks snappiest on a man who has a tanned or ruddy complexion. Fair-haired men look best in a medium to darker shade of brown. Charcoal brown, the most sophisticated of the brown suit family, looks best on men who have black, gray, or white hair. And since the color brown runs the gamut from tan to charcoal brown, you have a king-sized selection of shirt colors to wear. With a tan suit, consider shirts in soft shades of pink, blue or green. Light gray and blue shirts work well with all brown suits. As for ties, gray, green, olive, and gold all look handsome with a brown suit; solid black knits and black and white ties look particularly dashing with a tan suit. Especially smart, too, are a pale pink shirt and dark red tie worn with a tan suit. Tan and ivory ties are great-looking sartorial companions for suits in the darker shades of brown.

A gray suit in medium to darker shades is most flattering to men with blond, gray, or white hair. If you have a tanned or ruddy complexion, you can wear any shade of gray. White, pink, blue, pale yellow, and pale olive shirts look particularly nifty with a gray suit. A gray shirt with a gray suit? Avoid the combination if you have gray hair. In fact, skip it altogether unless the gray of the shirt is lighter than the gray of the suit and really offers a striking contrast. When it comes to ties, be as uninhibited as you like in the color department, ruling out only a solid gray tie of the same tone as your suit.

A green suit is no longer the rarity it once was, and since there are so many shades of green available in suits these days, any man can look good in a green suit. The suble gray-green shade known as loden green is very easy to wear, and as a bonus, it adapts extraordinarily well to all sorts of shirt and tie color combinations—shirts of light blue, gray-blue, pale green, bone, clear yellow, white, and ivory; ties of dark blues, dark greens, and dark reds. Olive green comes in a wide variety of tones, so if your hair is white or gray, avoid the lighter tones of olive. The dark shade called hunter green looks handsome on a man with gray or white hair and marries well with shirts of tan, beige, clear yellow, lemon yellow, ivory, white, and any shirt with stripes of pink and white or strawberry and white. As for ties, a hunter green suit looks best with solid color light green, light green and white, or light green and red striped ties. Best tie colors for an olive green suit: yellow, green, brown, tan, gold, gray, rust, and maroon.

Pattern-on-pattern fashion shouldn't faze any man in these liberated times. Mix patterns well, and you achieve the air of casual elegance that's the mark of a well-dressed man. For starters, there are a couple of basic truths to bear in mind.

1. *Patterns differ when it comes to strength.* Big bold checks, for instance, pack more wallop than minute checks, so make sure that one pattern is more subdued than the other.

2. *Color affects patterns.* A shirt with a light blue stripe, for instance, can handle a tie with more pattern than a shirt with a hot pink stripe.

Now here are some guidelines. Be brave and experiment.

	Shirt	*Tie*
SOLID COLOR SUIT		
	Solid color	Anything except solid color
	Narrow stripes	Anything except stripes of the same width as the shirt stripes
	Checks	Solid color Under-the-knot designs Panel designs Wide stripes

	Shirt	Tie
STRIPED SUIT	Solid color	Anything
	Narrow stripes if suit stripe is strong, wide stripe if suit stripe is muted	Anything except stripes
BOLD PLAID SUIT	Solid color	Solid color Under-the-knot designs Panel designs Wide stripes Small all-over figures Polka dots
	Narrow stripes	Solid color Under-the-knot designs Panel designs Wide stripes Small all-over figures Polka dots
MINIATURE PLAID SUIT	Solid color	Solid color Under-the-knot designs Panel designs Narrow or wide stripes Small all-over figures Bold patterns Subtle polka dots
	Narrow stripes	Solid color Under-the-knot designs Panel designs Wide stripes Small all-over figures Bold patterns Subtle polka dots

	Shirt	Tie
CHECKED SUIT		
	Panel designs	Solid color
	Wide stripes	Under-the-knot designs
HERRINGBONE SUIT		
	Solid color	Solid color
		Narrow or wide stripes
		Bold patterns
		Small all-over figures
		Checks and plaids
	Narrow stripes	Solid color
		Wide stripes
		Bold patterns
		Small all-over figures
		Checks and plaids
	Checked	Solid color
		Wide stripes

AFTER DARK

The tuxedo, or dinner jacket, first appeared on the scene one night in 1886, when a fashion maverick by the name of Griswold Lorillard wore it to a white-tie-and-tails autumn ball in exclusive Tuxedo Park, New York. No one took liberties with the tuxedo, however, until the 1920s, when the Prince of Wales, trend setter *extraordinaire* and later the Duke of Windsor, bypassed the traditional black tuxedo for one in midnight blue. But the tinkering with tradition stopped there, and as late as 1935 *Esquire* magazine was commenting on the fact that fashions in formal evening clothes change very little.

But today a man may turn up for a semiformal occasion dressed in a black velvet blouson or a double-breasted navy blazer worn with classic tuxedo trousers and be considered perfectly correct. Still, tradition counts for something even these days, and there are some formal occasions when there's positively no room for deviations from the norm. Correct is *correct*. Formal evening wear means "white tie," no ifs, ands, or buts.

For those relatively few white occasions—benefit dinners, debu-

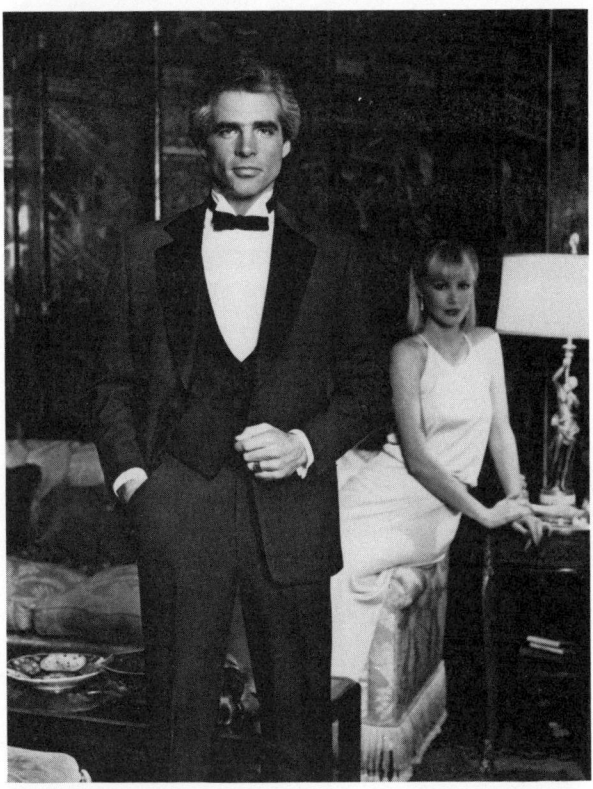

TUXEDO BY LORD WEST.

tante parties, balls, and official public affairs—here are the hard-and-fast dress rules.

Wear a tailcoat of either black or midnight blue (once upon a time only black was considered correct) with satin or grosgrain silk facings on the lapels. (Tails should extend only a fraction of an inch below the bend of the knee in back.) Trousers must be of the same fabric as the coat, with a single pleat or no pleats at all at the waistband. The obligatory white piqué waistcoat can be either single- or double-breasted, the wing-collared shirt with white piqué bosom, should have an inch of shirt cuff showing, and the butterfly bow tie is also white piqué. Black patent leather shoes may be either a pump, a laced shoe, or a slip-on. A white pocket handkerchief is preferably silk, and with white tie—and only with white tie—the handkerchief should have several of its points showing (triangle fold, this is called). Cuff links are either white pearl or a semiprecious stone, and if you wear a wristwatch, see that the band is either black leather or black suede.

Semiformal evening wear means black tie. Here a man has some

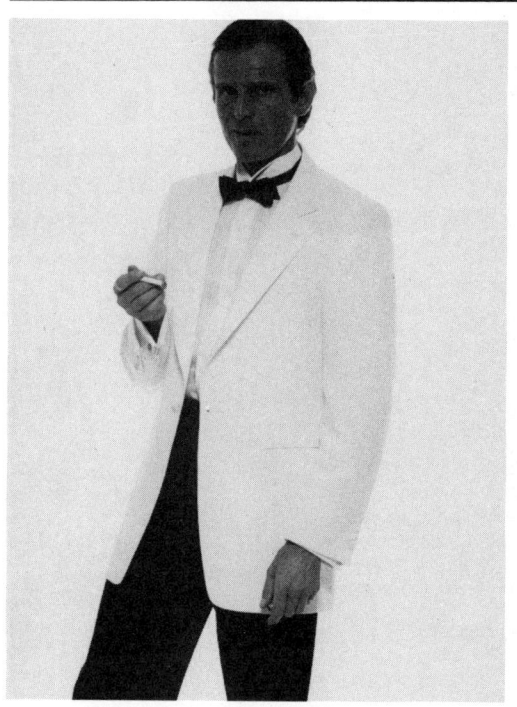

BILL BLASS FOR AFTER SIX.

choice as to what he can wear and still be correct. For example, a black or midnight blue dinner jacket is still expected September to May, but come the summer months you can, if you wish, wear a white dinner jacket or something colorful—pastels, stripes, even vibrant colors are acceptable nowadays. But I think most men recognize the fact that there's something decidedly impressive about a white shirt worn with a black or midnight blue tuxedo with satin lapels (the grand old wing-collared shirt has made an impressive comeback for semiformal wear in its new soft and washable guise. I think it looks terrific, but there's one thing to bear in mind: Its crisp lines are just not compatible with even a faintly jowly profile). The butterfly bow tie is black or midnight blue depending on the dinner jacket (in the summer if you wear something more colorful, just make certain that your bow matches your waistcoat or cummerbund). As for the aforementioned white shirt, it may be pleated or tucked and, of course, has French cuffs. Cuff links may be black onyx, smoked or black pearl, gold, or semiprecious stones in dark blue or dark red. Shoes may be black patent leather or polished calfskin, although I recommend you think in terms of black patent leather dancing pumps with traditional grosgrain bows or a two-eyelet patent leather oxford; both styles are correct for both black-tie and white-tie occasions. There have been times when some misguided men took to wearing red wool socks with their tuxedoes, but I haven't seen any of that nonsense lately; black unribbed socks are *the* socks to wear. When you're all dressed, tuck a handkerchief into your breast pocket—it can be white, a solid color, or a paisley.

Now a word about how to insert your pocket handkerchief. *Don't* use the triangle fold—it looks much too formal for a black-tie occasion—and the straight fold (a narrow band of handkerchief showing) is old-fashioned and monotonous-looking. Use the *puff*, it looks smartly casual for the good reason that it is. All you do is take all four corners of the square, shake, fold, and insert it into your pocket.

Perhaps you'd like to wear a velvet dinner suit. No reason why you shouldn't, but along with a velvet suit comes a special set of fashion guidelines. First of all, the velvet dinner jacket should be in a subdued shade: deep navy, deep brown, deep green, or maroon. Your butterfly bow tie should also be in a deep shade harmonious with your suit. Socks should be either black or a deep solid color keyed to the color of your suit, while shoes should be patent leather and in a color compatible with your suit. As for shirt and jewelry, they should be the same as what you'd wear with a more conventional tuxedo.

SHOE TALK

It's estimated that Americans walk 3,000 miles a year. It doesn't make sense that a man scrimp when it comes to buying shoes because well-made shoes look better and last longer. Buy the best you can afford, and be a shrewd shopper. Know something about leather —more than just how it looks. For example. . . .

Side leather is most often used for shoes for the good reason that not only is it tough and durable, but it's also lightweight and has plenty of "give."

Calfskin, as the name suggests, is taken from calves and is a younger, highly elastic leather with a very smooth appearance. Not surprisingly, it costs more than other leathers.

Patent leather was once upon a time reserved for formal and semiformal wear because it easily wrinkled and cracked with wear. Not so today. Current patent leather is much more durable, and as a result, you see more and more patent leather being worn with business suits. A white patent leather slip-on makes a stylish summer shoe. And patent leather offers a bonus: Since this leather's been coated to give a permanent shine, to keep it looking great, all you need do is wipe it clean with a damp soft cloth or, if you prefer, invest in a bottle of a colorless cleaner and conditioner made especially for patent leather, not only to clean it but to keep the leather flexible. Never use petroleum jelly on patent leather; it gums it up and dulls the shine.

Suede is a finish rather than an actual leather. Elegant suede, like patent leather, needs no polishing. Brushing is all it needs, but beware of the small wire brushes being sold for suede shoes; they scratch the nap. Instead, use a small rubber brush with rows of compact rubber "teeth" that bring up the nap gently. An art gum eraser will also remove light dirt.

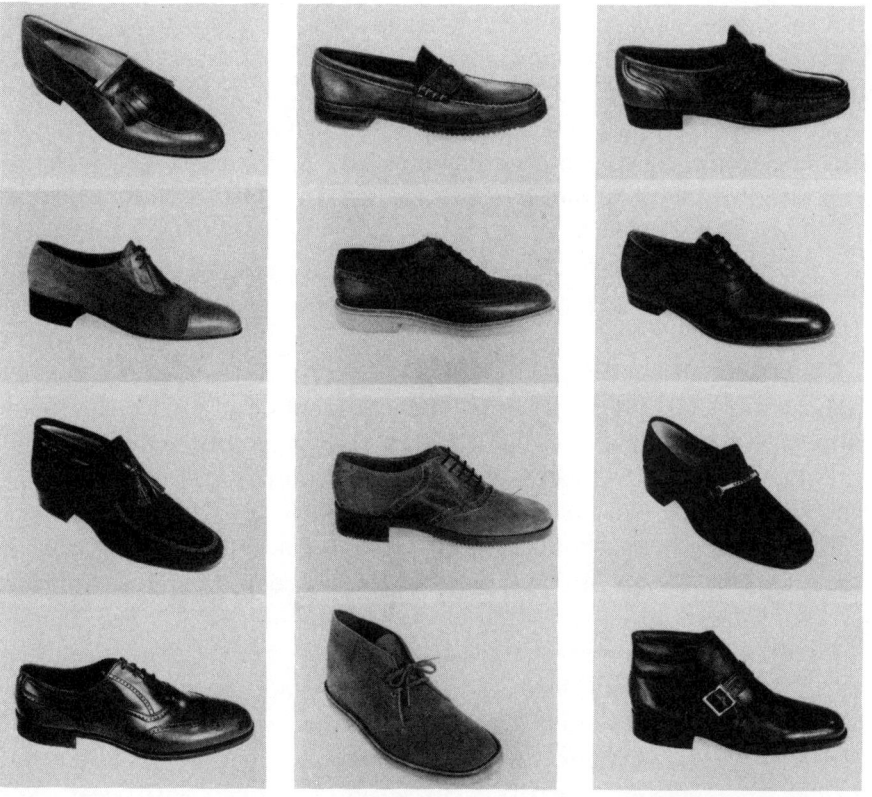

PHOTOS COURTESY OF THE FOOTWEAR COUNCIL.

Buckskin is a velvety soft leather with a suedelike finish. In brown or all white it makes a superior casual shoe.

Cordovan comes from the hindquarters of a horse, so it's not all that surprising, I suppose, that it's an extremely tough leather. One problem: It's hot on the foot since it isn't porous. On the plus side, however, cordovan takes a spectacular polish and is extraordinarily scuff-resistant.

Fashion Tips

If you're short, avoid a rounded or blunted toe; it makes a small foot look smaller. If you're tall and thin, steer clear of a very pointed toe.

For business wear, a laced shoe or a slip-on is correct, but tassel loafers are not. A decade ago an executive vice-president of a major blue-chip corporation, noting a young executive's tasseled loafers, remarked, "That fellow can't be very serious about his career." Antique thinking, I grant you, but still, the tassel loafer just never seems correct—too casual—in a business setting.

A heel higher than one and one-half inches is too high because body weight is tilted toward the toe area, thus pushing the toes into the front of the shoe.

Tips on Caring for Your Shoes

1. Thin and worn-out soles give little protection between you and the pavement, and put your metatarsal arch in jeopardy. Look at the sole, and feel it, too, by putting one hand inside the shoe and the other underneath. Compare it to a new shoe, and keep track of it, so that you can fix it before it wears too thin.

2. Run-down heels add to uneven walking patterns, which, in turn, increase unnatural pressure on the foot. As one calculatedly eccentric fashion pundit has put it: "A run-down shoe is the end of civilization." You get the point.

3. Inspect the inside of the shoe for lining wear. Toes can poke through. Rough-wearing interiors are hard on the skin of your feet and a breeding ground for germs. The pad covering the inner sole should be clean and smooth; replace it when it gets worn.

4. Shoe polish can keep your shoes looking like new. Use it regularly, and buff like crazy for a bright shine. There are liquids, foams, creams, and paste waxes, each polish having a particular quality. Foams and liquids cover scuffing well, creams clean and

soften the leather, and wax protects and polishes. Occasionally you may want to use them in combination.

5. Try never to wear a pair of shoes two days in a row. Give shoes a rest between wearings. They'll last longer that way because the inside lining is allowed to dry out. When shoes are worn steadily, foot moisture builds up inside the shoe, encouraging bacteria growth and material rot.

6. Put trees in the shoes you're not wearing. The purpose of a tree is to keep the shoe stretched out and in shape. There are wooden trees, but I prefer the metal ones; they leave more room inside the shoe and, consequently, air the shoe better.

7. Metal taps at the front underside of each shoe will protect the fronts from wearing out; rubber taps will do the same for heels.

8. Always use a shoehorn; using your finger, a ruler, or whatever else happens to be handy will crush the back of the shoe.

9. Since leather requires constant lubrication, be sure to polish shoes that haven't been worn for a while, that have been stored all summer, for example.

10. Avoid wearing suede shoes in rainy weather, when they can become permanently stained.

SOCK TALK

With the advent of the Peacock Revolution, men's hosiery kicked up its heels and lost its inhibitions. Result: more patterns, luscious colors. But socks still come in three lengths—anklet, mid-calf, and over-the-calf—and when you're wearing a business suit, there's only *one* length: over-the-calf.

The color of your socks should relate to your tie, not to your suit, but bear in mind that the size and color of their pattern are dictated by the suit you're wearing. In short, your suit wears the socks, the accessory, and not the other way around.

Don't be timid about wearing patterned socks with a business suit. But if your suit, shirt, and tie are providing you with pattern-on-pattern, you'd be wise to settle for solid color hose. In fact, they'll provide an interesting note of contrast.

Wool and cotton lisle are the best sock materials. Synthetic fiber socks simply aren't as absorbent as wool or cotton—unless they're *antistatic*. This special treatment is known as Endo-Stat, and when you read it on a label or hang tag, it means not only that the socks

DRESSING RICH

won't collect lint or have your trouser legs clinging to your socks but also that the socks will be more absorbent and, as a result, cooler to wear.

Socks may be either hand- or machine-washed. Use hot water for synthetics; warm water for wool or cotton. The latter should be hung to dry to avoid shrinkage.

HAT TALK

The derby is dead; the homburg is old hat. No matter. There are a lot of other styles, and men are wearing them. Why not? Hats are the finishing touch to a well-dressed appearance. There are a couple of other good reasons for wearing a hat. Our winters have been

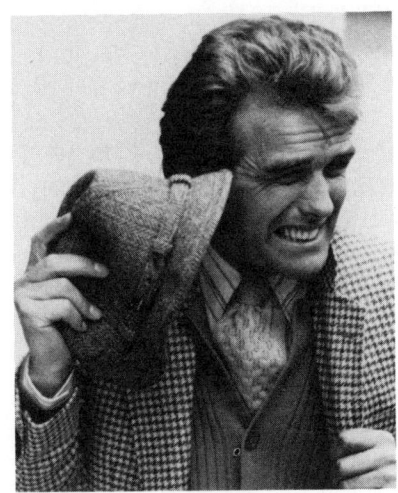

PHOTO COURTESY OF
J. P. STEVENS & CO., INC.

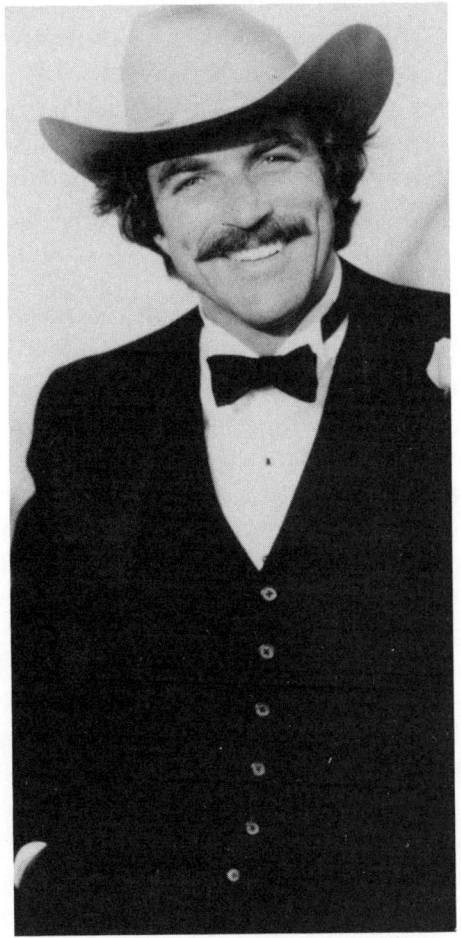

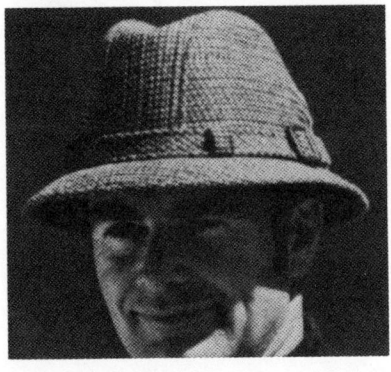

HAT BY KNOX.

PHOTO COURTESY OF REVLON.

getting increasingly arctic, and since about 40 percent of body heat escapes from the head, a hat is a very practical accessory; furthermore, a hat is a stylish cover for thin, tough-to-manage hair.

Today's hats have grown increasingly soft, comfortable, and, in some instances, even crushable, reminding me of a quote attributed to Fred Astaire to the effect that he will often take a brand-new hat and throw it up against the wall a few times to get the stiff, square newness out of it.

The cloth hat Rex Harrison made so popular in *My Fair Lady* is now more popular than ever, for nothing's softer, more comfortable, more crushable—or more adaptable. Wear it down all around or up in back; it's a true do-it-yourself hat. Popular, too, is the high, wide, and handsome western hat. Once upon a time it was strictly regional, and if you saw one on a man anywhere in the United States, you just assumed that he came from Marlboro Country. No more. Today he may be from New York, Chicago, or Little Rock, for the western influence is seen everywhere.

Few men can wear every hat style. Face shape and general physique are the determining factors. A short man, for example, can't carry a western hat. So when choosing a hat, stand in front of a full-length mirror. Meantime, let the following rules serve as a guide.

The slender face takes a well-tapered crown with a rather narrow brim. If you are short and slender, avoid too low a crown; if you are tall and slender, avoid too high a crown and too narrow a brim.

The plump face needs a full crown. The brim should be medium width and flat-set, rather than sharply rolled. If you are short and plump, avoid too wide a brim; if you are tall and plump, combine the full crown with a moderately wide flat-set brim.

The square face asks for a full crown with a medium brim. But a broader brim may suit, depending on your height.

Tips on Caring for Your Hat

1. Start off right by putting it on your head properly. Hold the brim in the front and back with both hands, and place the hat on your head at a slight angle to the left or to the right.

2. It's a myth that rain harms felt. When you are caught in a downpour, simply put your hat on a shelf to dry (not near a radiator), with the sweatband turned out. When it's dry, brush it with a soft-bristled brush.

OUTERWEAR

There are three coats which are now genuine fashion classics: the camel's hair polo coat, the British warm, and the chesterfield. They're still great buys. Have one of each, and you've got yourself a *super* coat wardrobe.

Camel's hair is a lightweight, soft, comfortably warm wool. Add to that the fact that its blond-tan shade is extraordinarily flattering, and you've got yourself quite a coat. It was popularized in the 1920s by visiting British polo players, who wore it between chukkers and after matches. Back then the classic polo coat was a six-button double-breasted model with half belt. Today a camel's hair wraparound with no buttons and a tied belt is deservedly popular, but it's scarcely for the man with an expanding waistline.

The British warm is another fashion classic of the same era, tracing its origin back to the taupe World War I British officer's coat, and it hasn't changed much in the intervening decades. Almost all these subtly shaped coats still carry their epaulets, though the original and very serviceable melton cloth has now been joined by a variety of fabrics, notably cashmere and cavalry twill, a very tough hard-finished worsted.

The chesterfield, named for a nineteenth-century earl of Chesterfield, is plain-backed and slightly shaped and has a velvet or a self-collar. It's usually in dark gray, blue, or black, but it's being seen in a variety of shades of brown, too. The black chesterfield offers an additional fashion bonus in that it can double as a very correct overcoat for formal and semiformal evening wear.

How to Care for a Wool Coat

1. Brush it with a soft brush after each wearing before hanging it in the closet.

2. A wet wool coat should never be put in the closet but should be hung up to dry—away from direct heat.

3. When putting it away for the summer, first clean it, and then store it in a garment bag containing mothballs.

How to Care for a Leather Coat

1. Avoid using the saddle soap and polish you use for leather shoes and boots because they can discolor a leather coat. Instead, spot clean by using a damp cloth, mild soap, and warm water. When

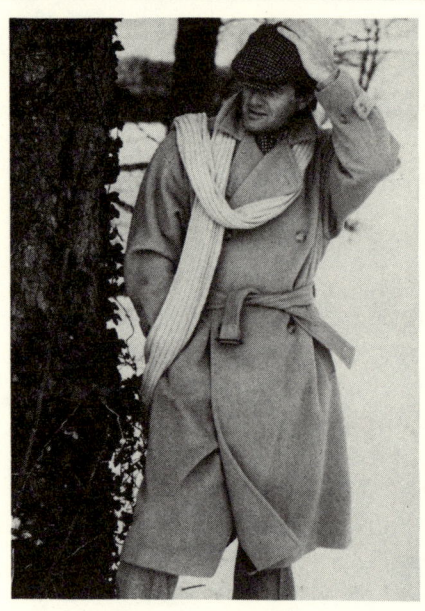

CAMEL HAIR COAT BY ALFRED DUNHILL OF LONDON.

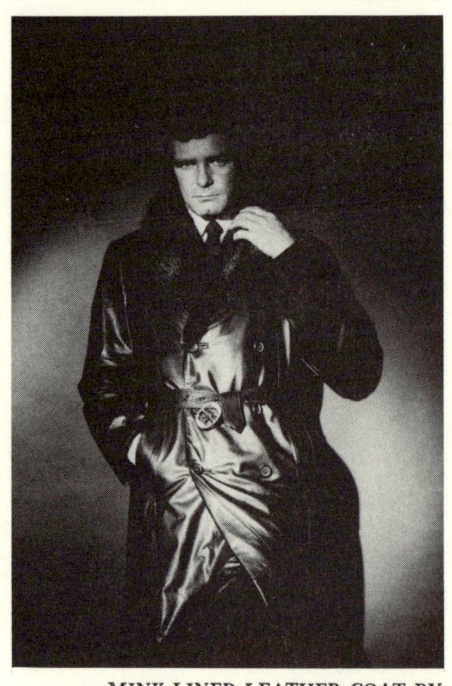

MINK-LINED LEATHER COAT BY ZILLI FOR PARVIZ.

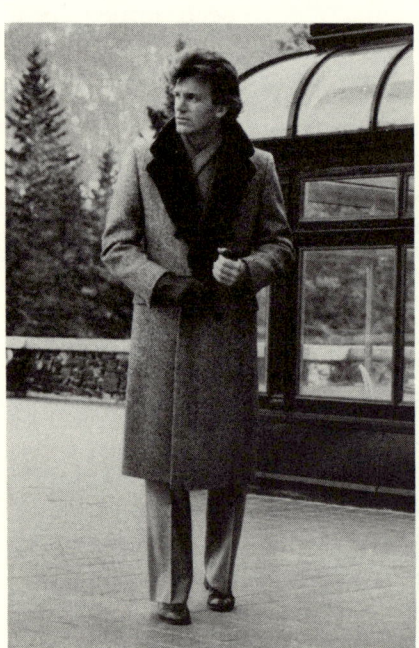

BILL BLASS FOR MALCOLM KENNETH.

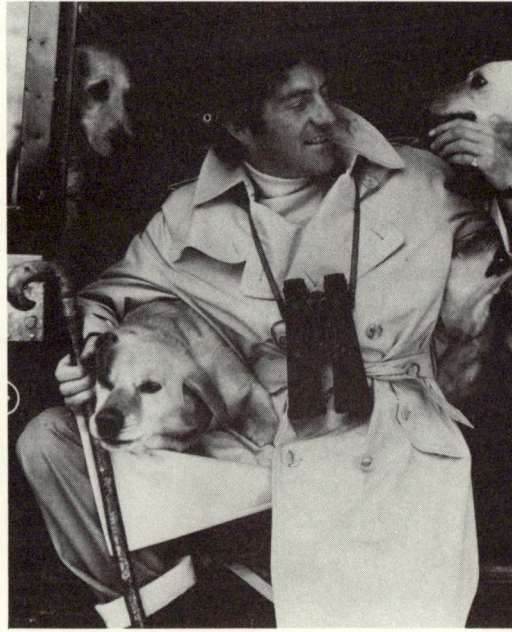

TRENCH COAT BY BURBERRY'S LTD.

the time comes for a complete cleaning, go to a cleaner who understands leather and uses a petroleum type of solvent that won't rob the leather of the oils that keep it supple.

2. Leather coats aren't designed for wet-weather wear because frequent exposure to rain will dry out the natural oils.

3. Come summer, put your leather coat in a cloth bag in a well-ventilated closet. A plastic bag is heat-making, and when temperature is humid, leather may mildew.

ROBE AND SLIPPERS

You may sleep in the buff or in a pair of silk pajamas. No matter. I still think you should treat yourself to a really fine robe and nifty slippers. I don't know of anything sartorially that does more to ease the stress and strain of modern living than to lounge around the house on, say, a Sunday in a monogrammed robe of silk, velour, camel's hair, cashmere, or flannel and a pair of velvet or patent leather house slippers. Expensive, but worth it.

JEANS

These have been a durable example of Americana ever since Levi Strauss cut the first pair back in 1850. They are described in the *Dictionary of American Slang* as "a pair of stiff, tight-fitting, tapered denim cowboy work pants, usually blue, with heavily reinforced seams and slash pockets." And so they are, but in the seventies designers latched on to jeans, and as a result, they're now available in everything from velvet to hopsacking, with the designer's own "brand" clearly in evidence.

Well, don't be intimidated into thinking that jeans are now the property of the compulsively trendy under-thirty crowd. We wore them first, and they're still a great fashion investment. Stay true to the classic blue jeans styling, and you can't go wrong. Avoid the stovepipe legs, the bell-bottoms, and all the other styling gimmicks. The blue denim jeans you wore way back when will never go out of style. Be an elegant classicist, and wear them with a button-down shirt and a great-looking sweater or sports jacket; that's the look that no one can carry off with the chic of the seasoned All-American Man. And should you need a role model before taking up jeans again, Cary Grant says, "Most of the time I walk around in jeans."

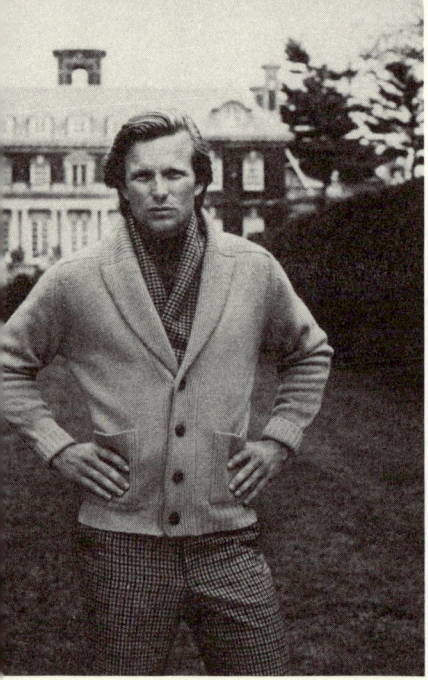

SWEATER BY LORD JEFF.

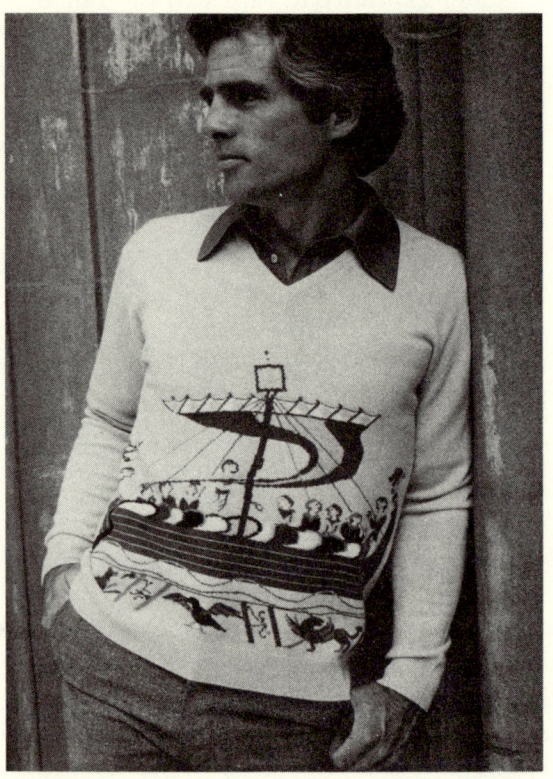

CASHMERE SWEATER BY PRINGLE OF SCOTLAND.

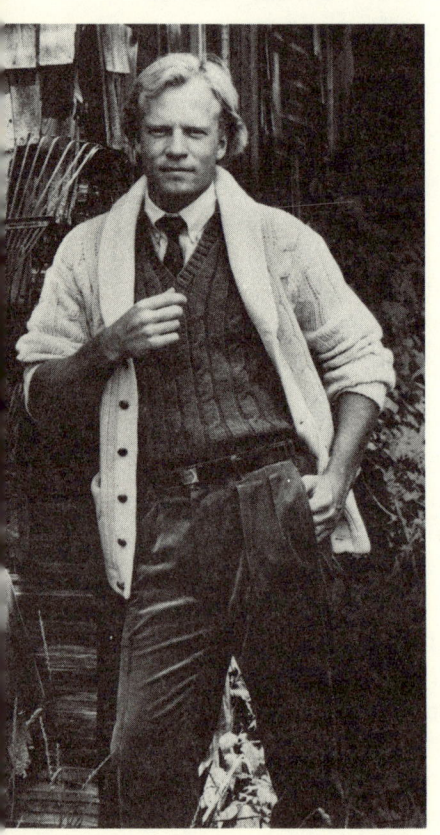

SWEATERS BY POLO.

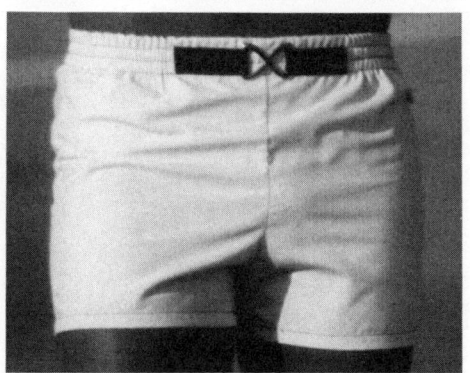

PHOTO COURTESY OF JANTZEN.

SWIMWEAR

It comes in a great variety—and so does the American physique. A well-tailored suit can conceal a multitude of flaws, but when a man —especially a mature man—slips into a swimsuit, he often requires a little camouflage.

So unless you've got an exercise program going that's really working for you, avoid the short-short trunks that rest on the hipbone and have square-cut legs. Most flattering to all types of physiques is the swimsuit modeled after the Bermuda walking short; it's extremely well tailored, and the extra length in the leg has a slimming effect. But this model's not for you if you're on the short side; the extra leg length tends to have a shortening effect. Boxer-type shorts styled like boxer undershorts are safe for any body type, but they certainly don't have much dash. An updated version of the old tank suit, on the other hand, has plenty of dash, but not for you if you're the least bit corpulent. As for the bikini—forget it.

FUR COATS

Esquire in November 1969 called its biggest fur coat feature to that date "The Fur Side of Paradise" and trumpeted the "renaissance of the fur-bearing male, who had been in retirement in the discreet decades since the coonskin coat was part of our collegiate culture." But by 1971 *Esquire* and every fashion magazine of stature were showing furs of nonendangered species or synthetic furs, as the

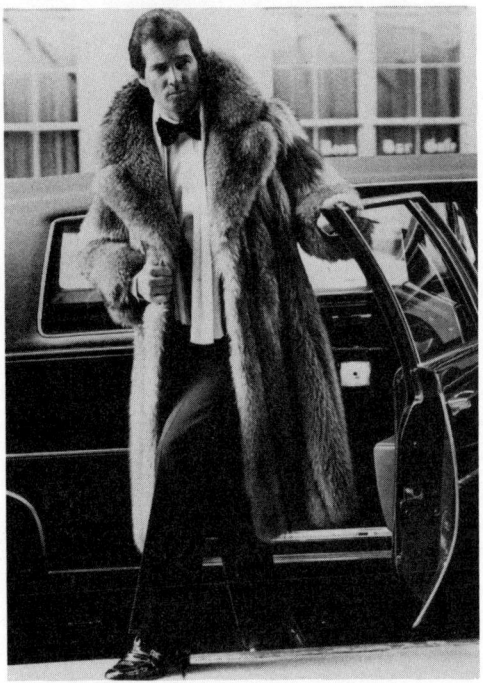

FISHER FUR COAT. PHOTO COURTESY OF
THE AMERICAN FUR INDUSTRY.

word "ecology" worked its way into the vocabulary of concerned Americans.

One successful designer of fur coats for men told me that "the more mature individual is the best customer for furs," accepting them as being as relevant to his life-style as, say, an expensive car. It's the career-oriented, affluent man who has been accounting for the bulk of fur sales at such first-class retail emporiums as Neiman-Marcus and Bergdorf Goodman, opting for such styles as a full-length flat-fur version of the classic Brooks Brothers belted-back topcoat. Flat furs look best on the mature man; the long-haired furs like coyote and raccoon look best on the under-thirty crowd.

Most men start first with a fur-lined or fur-trimmed coat before investing in a fur coat—a poplin trench coat with, say, an opossum lining or a dark blue wool with ample collar and cuffs of ranch mink.

Some man-made furs are great-looking, and their price tags are a fraction of what the genuine fur costs. Black Orlon, for instance, so closely resembles seal that only a seal could tell the difference.

Men appear to be more concerned with the durability of the furs they buy than women are. So for the record be advised that the longest-wearing fur is seal—up to twenty years—and a mink coat will look good for at least ten to fifteen years, depending, of course, on how well it's cared for. That includes storing the coat during the summer months in a fur vault, where it can be properly cleaned and mended, if necessary.

JEWELRY

Less is best. After the jangle of chains and pendants in the 1960s, it's nice to note that today's well-dressed man limits his jewelry to a few pieces of high quality. He wears no rings in general except a wedding ring—loving and traditional—and he wears a wristwatch with a strap in fine leather or suede or carries a wafer-thin pocket watch with an eighteen-karat gold chain. Should you hanker for a second ring, I suggest you make it a small gold crest ring designed to be worn on the little finger.

The ID bracelet or dog tag of World War II introduced American men to the idea of wearing bracelets, but few men seem to wear a bracelet with the casual elegance that's essential. Still, a thin gold chain bracelet can be a handsome accessory.

Giant-sized cuff links are in poor taste. The closer in size your cuff links are to the buttons on your shirt cuff, the better. I'm all for splurging when it comes to cuff links; they have a long life and are, I think, the most impressive piece of jewelry a man can wear. Consider an eighteen-karat gold ball, or an eighteen-karat gold knot —functional and elegant. If the price is prohibitive, there are knots of silky elastic cord that sell for a fraction of the price of gold (or silver) and are extremely attractive. But remember, don't mix your metals; it's all gold or all silver.

HOW TO REMOVE STAINS AND SPOTS

What's the difference between a stain and a spot? Well, a stain is a foreign substance that has made its way into the very fiber of the fabric, while a spot is a mark caused by food or liquid that surrounds the fiber of the fabric. Naturally, a spot is easier to deal with than a stain. There are nonliquid spot removers that don't leave a telltale ring. Should you use a cleaning fluid, however, let the spot dry before applying it, and have a clean white cloth be-

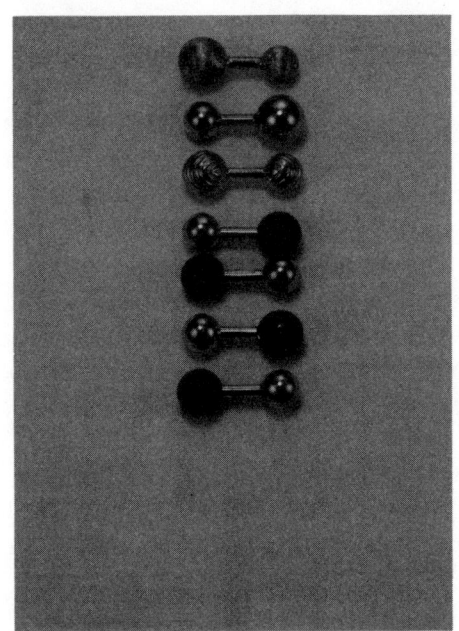

TIFFANY & CO.

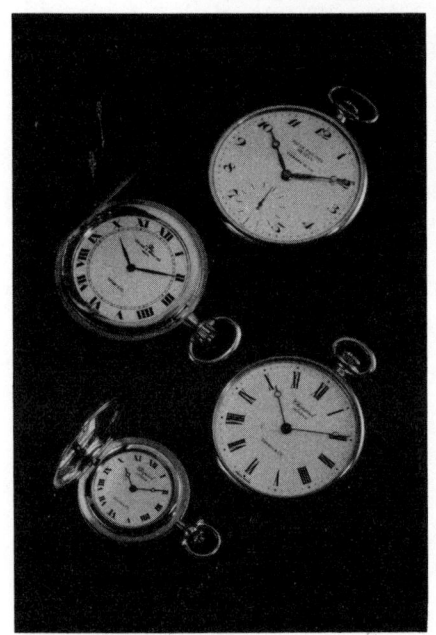

TIFFANY & CO.

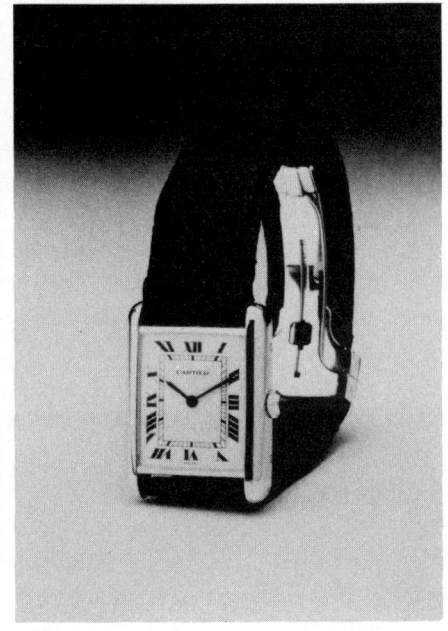

The famous Cartier "Tank" watch.

neath the stained area to sop up grime that may seep through to the other side.

When a stain is the problem, the sooner you get at it, the better your chance of removing it. That applies to any stain: greasy (butter, oil, ink); nongreasy (alcohol, catsup, coffee or tea without cream); or a combination of both (chocolate, ice cream, salad dressing).

Washing followed by warm-water rinsing will usually remove most greasy stains, provided the article is *washable*. For wash-and-wear or permanent-press fabrics, you may have to rub soap or detergent directly into the stain and let it stand for several hours before rinsing. If the article is *nonwashable,* sponge the greasy stain with a special grease solvent of the type used by dry cleaners, which is available at drugstores and supermarkets. Let it dry, and repeat if necessary. If a yellow stain remains, use a peroxide bleach.

TALKING SCENTS

Do you remember when the most fragrant thing a man could splash on himself was a little bay rum? Then, in 1965, *Life* magazine was reporting on "the big boom in men's beauty aids," and the following year a syndicated writer observed, "Already more dollars are spent for male fragrances in the United States than for female's." (You've come a long way, buddy.)

"As far as anyone can figure," *Life* went on, "the new era started in Paris and the Caribbean during the mid 1950's, when U.S. college men on vacation began buying a chic French cologne called Canoe (pronounced Can-oh-ay). . . . And when the boys came home wearing Canoe, the old man got adventuresome and tried a little too." Remarked one cosmetics industry executive at the time: "There is no reason why men shouldn't have the same emotional chords as women, just waiting to be plucked." Well, mine have been plucked, and I imagine yours have, too.

Of all the forms of men's fragrances, cologne is the most concentrated and lasting. It contains more alcohol and more perfume than an after-shave lotion and comes from any one of six basic aromas: citrus, flowers, wood, leather, spices, and tobacco. And it smells different on every man's skin because it's a question of the fragrance plus your individual body chemistry that makes it work or not work for you.

A dry skin needs a more generous splash of cologne than oily skin because it doesn't hold the fragrance as long. Be aware, too,

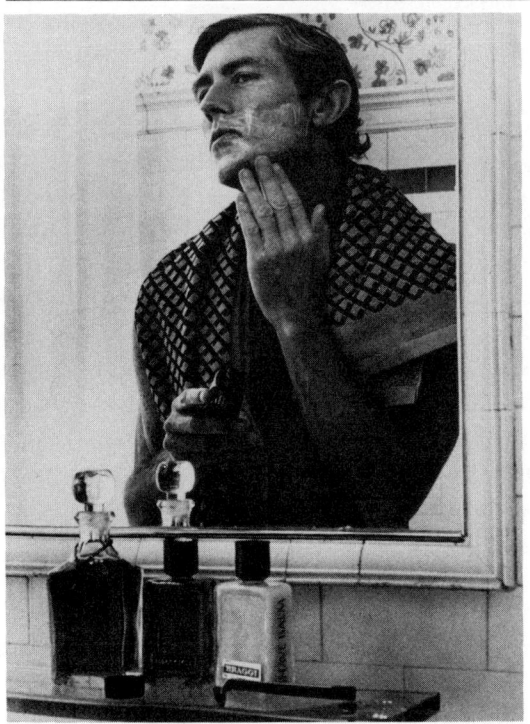

PHOTO COURTESY OF
MEN'S FASHION ASSOCIATION.

that the sense of smell (men over fifty are said to lose their ability to appreciate fully "smell sensation") isn't as keen in the morning as it is later in the day.

Wear a lighter scent in warm weather because heat intensifies fragrance. Save stronger fragrances for cooler weather.

Keep your colognes in a dark, cool place; long exposure to strong sunlight or extremes in temperature can disturb the balance of fragrance.

When shopping for a cologne, apply it directly to the skin. Use both wrists and palms of your hands as test areas. You can't get a true reaction to the fragrance from the bottle. Allow the heat of the body to develop the fragrance on your skin, and then sniff.

Assuming that you use both an after-shave lotion and a cologne, bear in mind that they should be compatible fragrances. The best way to assure this is to choose them from the same maker; as a result, both will have been derived from the same basic aroma.

PACKING IT IN

Here, too, less is best. Traveling light is the only way to travel; spend as little time as possible packing.

If necessary, start with a list so you won't put anything unessential in your luggage. Lay everything on your bed so that you can coordinate suits, ties, and shoes. Concentrate on items of apparel that can do double duty; a gray flannel suit and navy blazer, for example, add up to two outfits. Bring along a few ties that can go with everything; solid color knits are great, and furthermore, they don't wrinkle.

When possible, take luggage of feather-light nylon small enough to carry aboard the plane, and thus avoid the long wait at the other end.

When it comes to shirts, pack them flat, alternating the collars so that you'll have a compact rectangular package. Roll your socks tightly, and stuff them into your shoes, which you stash at the ends of soft luggage, at the bottom of the bag if it's a suitcase you're packing. Some men invest in a tie case, but I find it simple to roll my ties and use them to fill up corners of the bag. Roll belts, too, by sticking the end through the buckle and then curling the end inward.

How to Fold a Suit

For soft luggage

1. Spread the jacket out, lining down. Turn collar and lapels so that they're lying as flat as possible.
2. Keeping the sleeves flat, fold the shoulders toward the center of the back of the jacket until they meet.
3. Next, fold the lapels over the shoulders so that the lining is facing upward; then fold the jacket in half.
4. Lay the trousers out with the cuffs, creases, and waistband even. Place the folded jacket over the middle third of the trousers.
5. Now fold the bottom of the trousers over the jacket, and then fold the top of the trousers back over the entire bundle.

For a suitcase without hangers

1. Begin by buttoning the middle button of the jacket, then hold the jacket in both hands at each shoulder, and shake gently to remove the wrinkles.

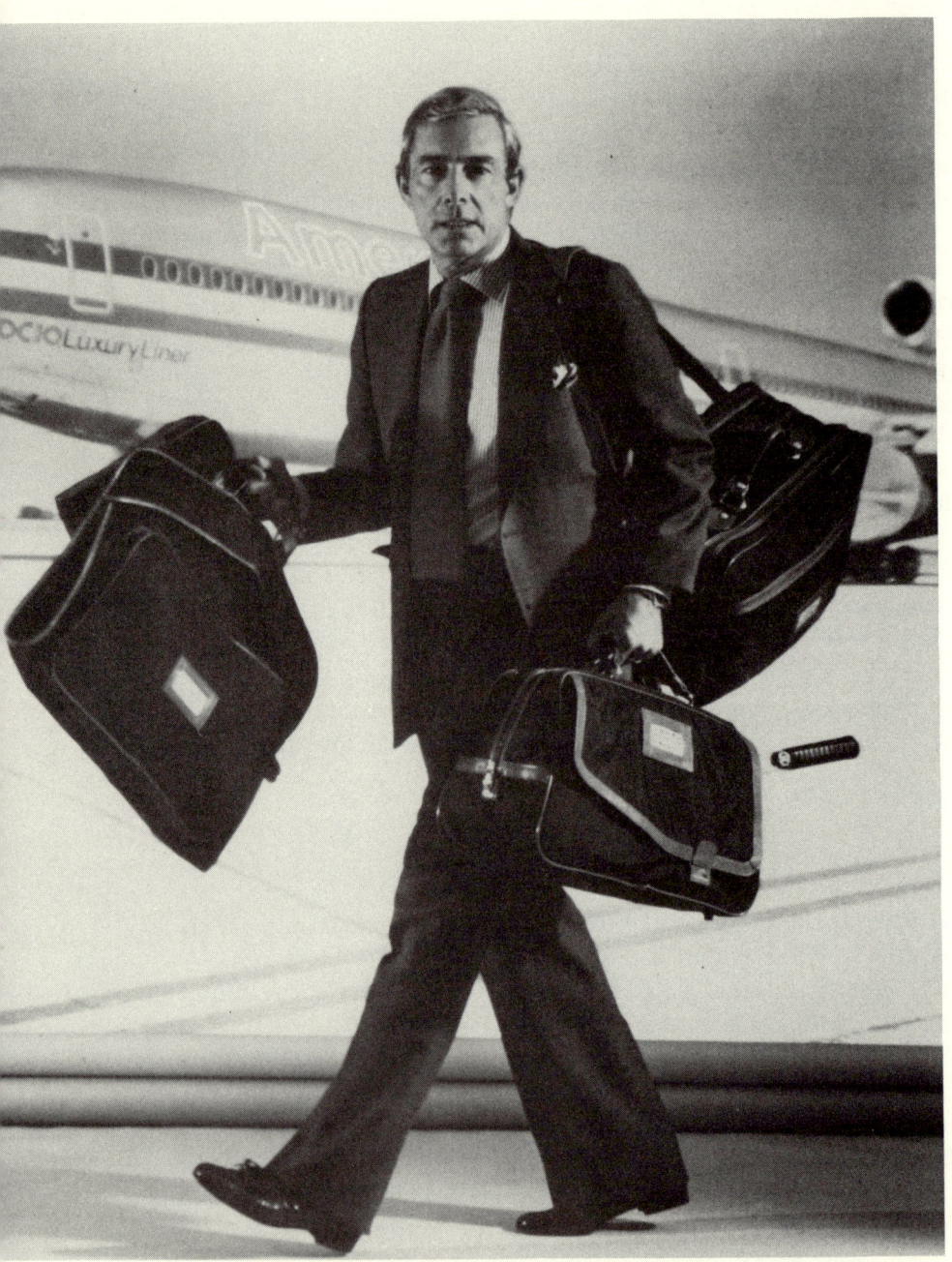

Luggage small enough to carry aboard the plane means no waiting at the other end. Here designer John Weitz carries his Weitz-designed luggage of feather-light nylon.

2. Next, place the jacket button side down on the bed, smoothing it out so that there's a minimum of wrinkles. If the pockets have flaps, make sure they are on the outside.

3. Fold each side of the jacket back from the shoulder to the bottom so that the edge of the sleeve at about the elbow is in line with the center seam in back of the jacket. Place a sheet of crumpled tissue paper lengthwise between the sleeves to minimize wrinkles.

4. Next, fold the jacket in half, and place it in the suitcase either vertically or horizontally depending on the shape of the suitcase.

5. To fold the trousers is easy. After brushing them, close the zipper, fold them in half, and place them at the bottom of the suitcase. If the waist measurement is more than average, fold the trousers over a vertical line at the seat; if your suitcase is relatively small, it may be necessary for you to fold the trousers twice. The suit jacket is placed above the trousers.

Final note: Unpack as soon as you reach your destination. Minor wrinkles can be steamed out by hanging the garment in the bathroom while running a hot shower.

A GALLERY OF MEN WHO LOOK AND FEEL LIKE A MILLION

Hardy Amies

Born 1909

It was in 1969 in London that I first met Hardy Amies. He was sixty years old at the time and looked forty. When I saw him again, ten years had passed, we were in New York City, and he had aged. He looked a youthful fifty.

By his own admission, he has shrunk. "I was six feet, but now I'm five feet ten and a half inches. We all shrink as we age," he says. "I know it's true, for I've had the X rays on my back."

A reporter once referred to him as "the popular idea of an Englishman—tall, fair and flat." A female reporter for *The New York Times* has called him "the world's most handsome royal dressmaker." True enough, but then how many royal dressmakers are there? Amies has been doing a third of Queen Elizabeth's wardrobe for the past twenty-five years, having started designing for her when she was Princess Elizabeth. "I've gone right through the reign," he says.

But so far as America is concerned, men are his customers, and his line of men's clothes is sold from coast to coast. In 1961 Amies was the first in England to start designing for men. Eight years later, the Amies men's fashion show I attended in New York opened with a bang. Actually, it was the music of the Grenadier Guards, and the models, four brought from London and eight Americans, came in all together in military-looking overcoats, carrying their umbrellas like rifles. "I like to dance on the fine line of being far out," says Amies.

"I weigh a hundred seventy and should like to be half a stone lighter—that's seven pounds—but then people say I look gaunt. So I feel well and I look well at a hundred seventy. I get very agitated if it gets above that. I'm a great believer in fasting—even a week's fasting. I mean absolutely no food at all, absolutely nothing. It's not difficult. The point? A total change of metabolism. I should like to do it once perfectly every six months. How often I do do it has to do with how much time I have at my disposal. I don't

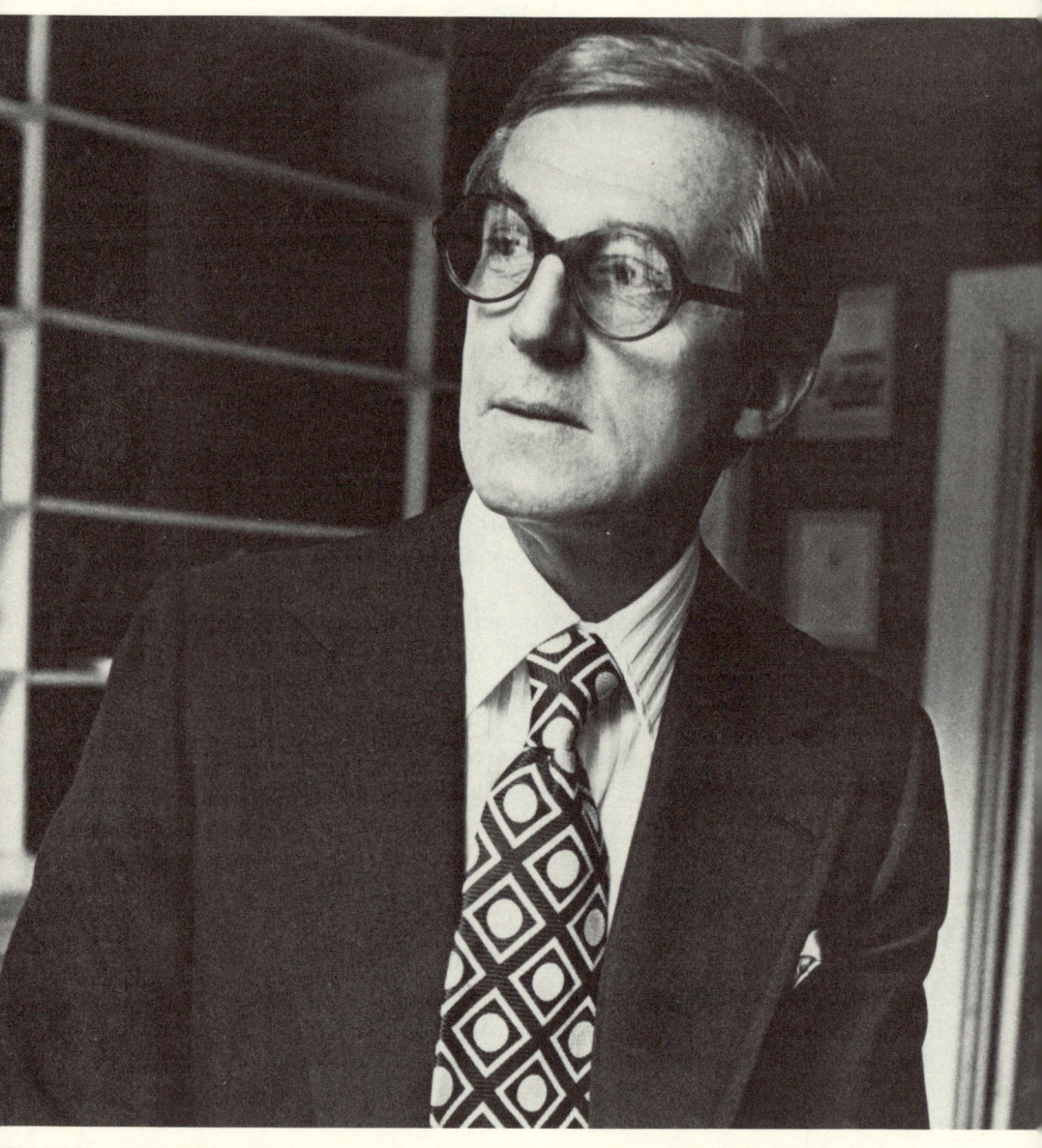

think you can do it in your own household. My doctor runs a clinic in the country outside London.

"What is so extraordinary about it is that you simply do not feel hungry. The great enemy of the whole thing is boredom. You see, you'd be amazed at how much time is taken up with meals. How the meal cuts up the day! My doctor would like you for the first twenty-four hours to stay in bed, to have nothing in your room. It's terribly austere. You're not allowed a radio, television, a book, *anything*. It so happens (don't laugh) that I do quite fine needlepoint, and so I do my needlepoint, and after that first day, I go for walks. Certainly there's no feeling of weakness whatsoever. It's staggeringly beautiful countryside on the border of Kent—beautiful moors, heather—and I walk for about an hour. When the fasting is over, it's very important that you resume eating the right foods in small amounts."

When in his native London, Amies walks two miles across Hyde Park to his business located in a Georgian mansion on Savile Row. When he's in New York City, he manages to get out and walk for at least a half hour no matter how busy he is. "I chose my apartment for its proximity to Central Park. My theory is that a walk should be upon the earth and with the trees. I think you've got to be in touch with the earth.

"I try to play tennis at least once a week. I have a country place seventy miles from London, near Oxford, near the source of the Thames. I have a tennis court there.

"I don't drink liquor; I drink wine. I'm a great bed-goer. Five hours' sleep is perfect for me, but then I like an hour in the afternoon; a nap after lunch is very important—even for twenty minutes. I work on the Churchillian principle, and that is that you should take all your clothes off; it gives you an immediate feeling of relaxation. I'm a morning person—up at six-thirty—and that's why I need the second breath of the nap.

"I'm very interested in cooking, but I don't overeat. I think commercialized white bread is one of the sins of progress. I have an old stove in my country cottage, and I'll make bread for a week and store it in the deepfreeze."

Amies is convinced that 75 percent of men don't sensibly plan their clothes buying and are color-blind as well. "They don't buy a suit with any idea of the shirt and tie they'll wear with it. I think that's a terrible mistake. And they always seem to forget the relationship of color to their own coloring. I have blue eyes, and I know blue is flattering to me because I also have fair skin. And speaking of skin, I use a regular safety razor and soap and water—nothing else. I don't like the feel of anything else on my face."

Meantime, at seventy, Hardy Amies is preparing to branch out "into household things: bed linens, kitchen linens, and things like that. I'm always thinking ahead. You have to in the fashion business, you know. I always see a new year shaping up."

Warren Anderson
Born 1921

Shortly before World War II a big towheaded teenager named Warren Anderson worked a couple of summers as lifeguard on one of Long Island's South Shore beaches. Every day it was like a Norman Rockwell magazine cover come to life: the little boys hanging around his station, waiting for the time he'd dive into the waves for some exercise, and their teenaged sisters hanging around, hoping he'd notice them. My family had a beach house there and one summer we had a new lifeguard. The big towhead had gotten a football scholarship to Colgate and no doubt a better-paying summer job.

Today Warren Anderson is president of Union Carbide and operates out of an executive suite hung with modern paintings and a white hard hat with his name stenciled on it. His hair is steel gray, but he still has the rugged physique of an athlete.

"I used to work out on a trapeze and parallel bars," he says. "And I like squash, but moving around the world so much on business gets me away from it." What regular exercise he gets now boils down to a fifteen-minute regimen of stretching exercises. "A mishmash of my own picked up through life; some were part of calisthenics before football playing, for example. And I walk every chance I get—walk fast."

A former beer drinker ("I grew up in a background where you might enjoy a can of beer before a meal"), he switched to bourbon early in his business career. "I was on the road for the company, and I ordered a beer at the bar of the Brown Hotel in Louisville, Kentucky, and the bartender said to me, 'Son, you're in bourbon country.' I like bourbon. Don't know whether that's good or bad. Anyway, I leave my drinking for cocktail parties on weekends."

He has a summer place now on Long Island's South Shore not far from where he used to be the lifeguard. He tends his own garden there. "Climbing up into a tall maple, I find I get a little more tired than I used to." And that's about the only sign of aging this boss of a $7.9 billion industrial corporation has noticed.

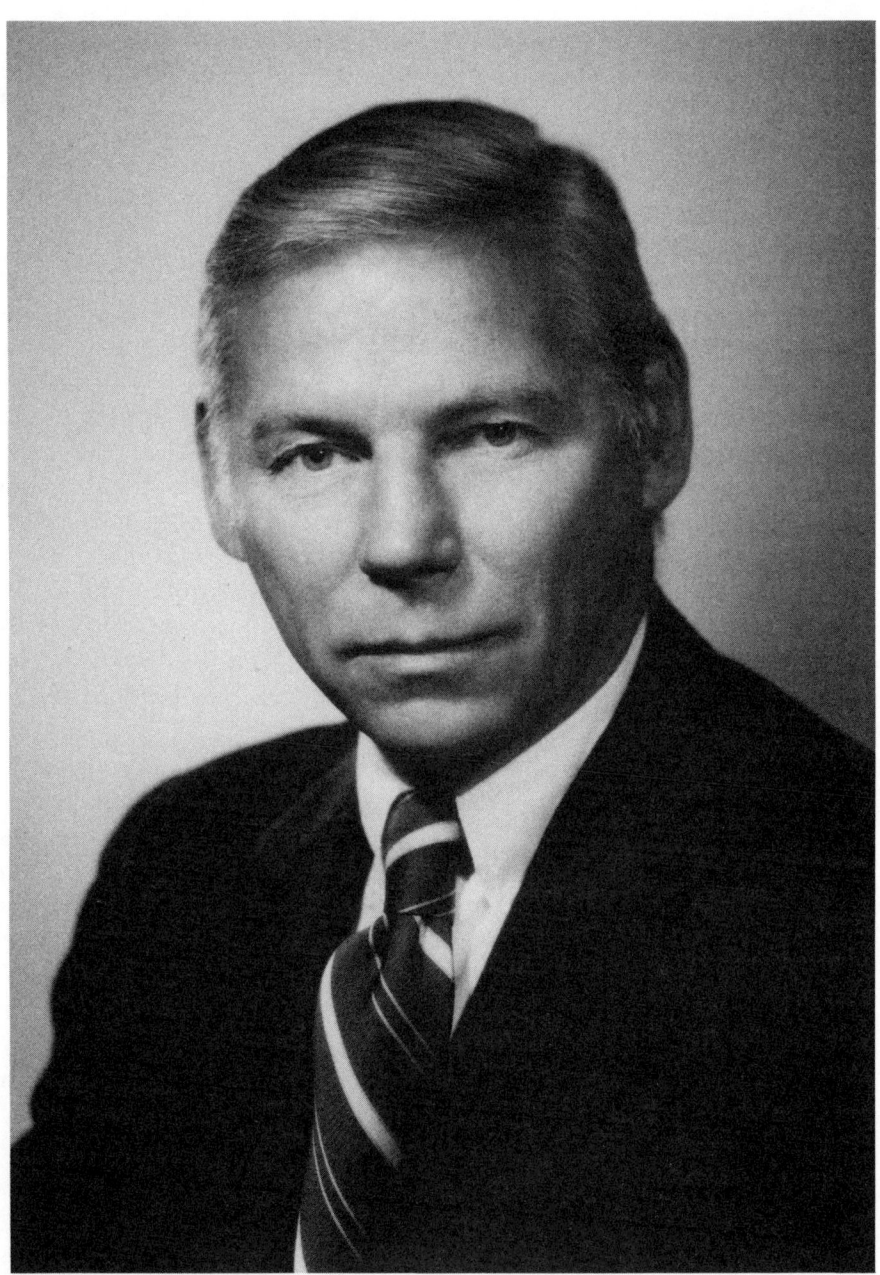

PHOTO BY FABIAN BACHRACH.

Bill Blass
Born 1922

"I wish someone would say something rotten about me," designer Bill Blass said last year at a dinner-dance reception at which he was given yet another creative award to add to his collection. There were 220 guests in attendance, but not one of them could think of anything rotten to say about him. For Blass, the sole owner of Bill Blass Ltd., is the good guy of the fashion world. He is also one of the richest, having expanded his talents to include not only menswear and women's wear but luggage, table linens, sheets and towels, an automobile, and, most recently, perfume.

The former high school football player from Fort Wayne, Indiana, went into menswear in the early sixties to supply clothes for the man over thirty who he thought had been neglected by the Peacock Revolution. He made his first impact via "bold patterned suits that would make him feel young."

Slouching comfortably in a chair in his New York office, the sleeves of his blue button-down shirt rolled up to the elbows, he looks relaxed and, as always, good-natured. "I work at it," he says. "I've really learned to relax in the last ten years. I don't get excited, I allow enough time to make planes, and I no longer have partners. I have found out that I have to do things my way. I have twenty-five licensees, and I personally get involved in everything. Fortunately I have high energy. Work stimulates me. I guess I've unconsciously weeded out people that chafe. It's better that way."

Blass doesn't think we'll see another men's fashion revolution for perhaps another 100 years. "Of course, that's too vast a prophecy," he concedes, but says that in his opinion "the sixties add up to an unfortunate period for men. It was okay for the young, but now they, too, are dedicated followers of the conservative in dress, and for that I'm thankful. Anyway, the United States is a very conservative nation—the most conservative.

"One dresses for his way of life," he says, "but regardless of lifestyle, anyone is not well dressed if too coordinated, too thought out or well matched."

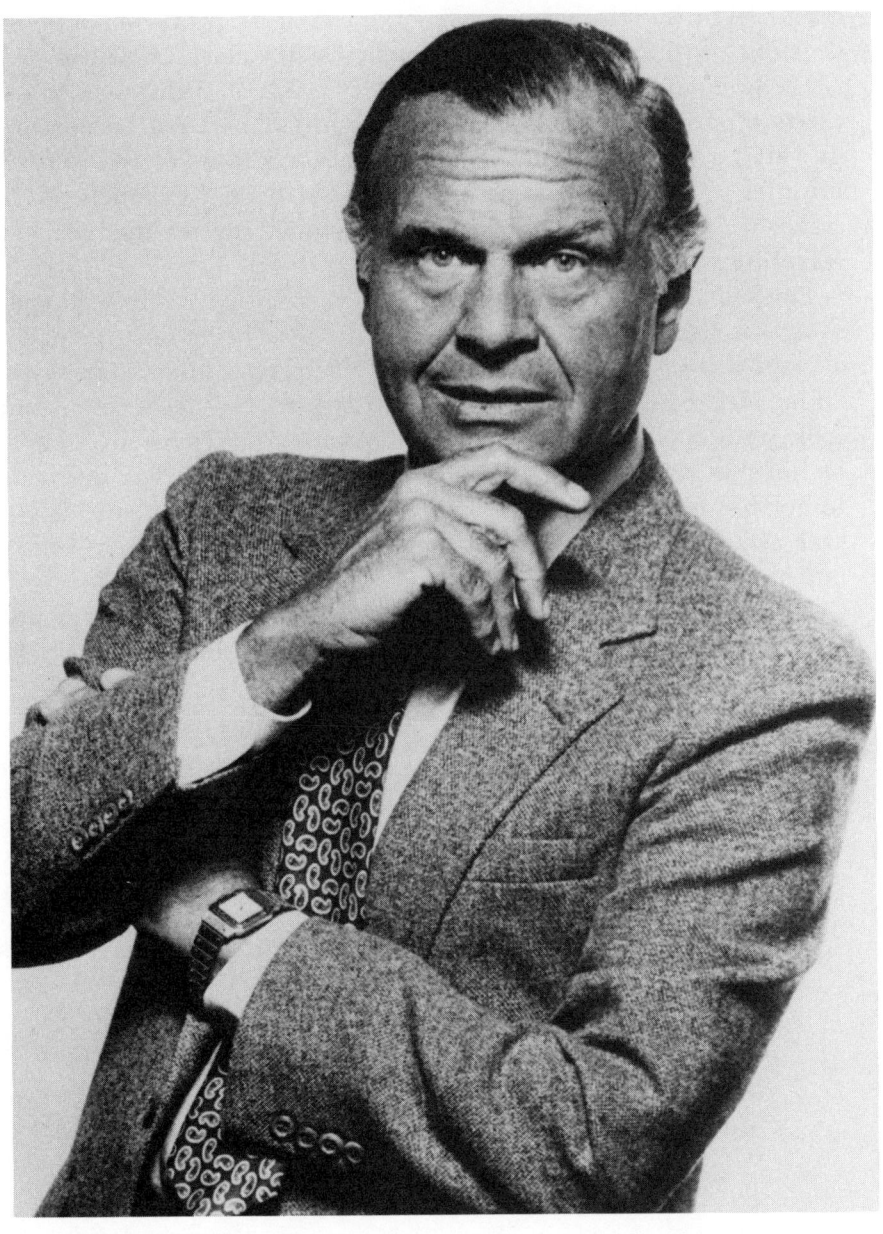

Blass also thinks that "men in America tend to be overweight, and to make matters worse, they wear clothes that are too big for them. Ill-fitting clothes are one of the biggest problems, and so is dressing youthfully when you're past the first flush of youth."

He walks home from his office every evening, a distance of some thirty blocks, and at his country place in Connecticut he does a lot of walking weekends with his dogs. "I also try to do fifteen to twenty minutes of exercise at home, too. I say *try to* . . . so much business travel is a deterrent. Most men, me included, aren't inclined when traveling to do exercises in hotels."

For years Blass spent $2,000 per week for two weeks at a spa in southern California, where recently he has been noting that the average age of the men is consistently getting younger. He reasons, "The successful man in business realizes to be successful he must look well, stay trim. That means he must know how to take care of his skin, his hair, et cetera." But recently Blass has decided to forgo the yearly visit to the spa. He'll stay fit without outside help. One can get too dependent on a spa, he says, and between visits get out of shape.

Has Bill Blass any vices? He smokes four packs of cigarettes a day. Will he give up smoking? "No," he says firmly, but with a smile.

Jeffrey Butler

Born 1939

As founder, publisher, chairman, president and sole stockholder of the East/West magazine network, Jeff Butler—according to *Time* magazine—"rules the friendly skies of in-flight magazines . . . with slick, thick, technicolor magazines throbbing with lively articles." He established his corporation in 1969 when the airline he was serving as public relations director (among his accomplishments he'd outfitted its stewardesses in tangerine-colored hot pants) balked at his plan to publish an in-flight magazine for an investment of $250,000. Today, his Los Angeles-based firm publishes magazines for ten airlines. And Jeff Butler is a millionaire with a fifteen-room home on the West Coast commanding an unobstructed view of the San Bernardino Mountains on one side and the Pacific Ocean on the other, and a duplex condominium in New York with a view of the Hudson River to the left and the East River to the right. Says Butler, "My wife is always kidding me that I don't feel comfortable in a house unless the view resembles the one out an airplane window."

He chose southern California as his base for several reasons, not the least of which is that "after four years with the army in Hawaii, you get spoiled when it comes to climate, and I felt southern California had the closest to the ideal climate," that is, one that enables him to swim in his pool every morning. "Swimming's my saving grace," he says. "It gets my circulation going." He weighs the same trim 168 pounds he did back in the days he was earning a baccalaureate degree in marketing at the University of Illinois.

When not in California, Butler travels around to East/West's twelve offices across the country. As a result, "most of the time I live in wool gabardine that tends to go anywhere in any climate." He seldom wears a hat when he's on the West Coast, but when he's in a blustery city he favors a soft, unconstructed felt with a fairly broad brim.

He washes his hair and uses eyedrops every day in recognition of the fact that his daily swim exposes him to the polluting effect of chlorinated water. He smokes about a pack of cigarettes a day, and he fights this other form of pollution with a daily intake of 2,000 mgs of vitamin C.

Sitting behind a $12,000 mahogany desk that spent one hundred of its two hundred and fifty years in residence at London's No. 10 Downing Street, the king of his own high-flying empire says that his thirty-seventh birthday impressed upon him, and not unpleasantly, that "my feeling of youth had pretty much left me. I was no longer feeling immature in the business world, which I was when I started my firm at twenty-nine. I had attained a level of inner confidence at last. And now that I'm into my forties, I have what I call an energy conservation approach to living. I see to it, for example, that I get seven hours' sleep every night. No more staying out and dancing until three in the morning—though I'm convinced I could still do it if I wanted to."

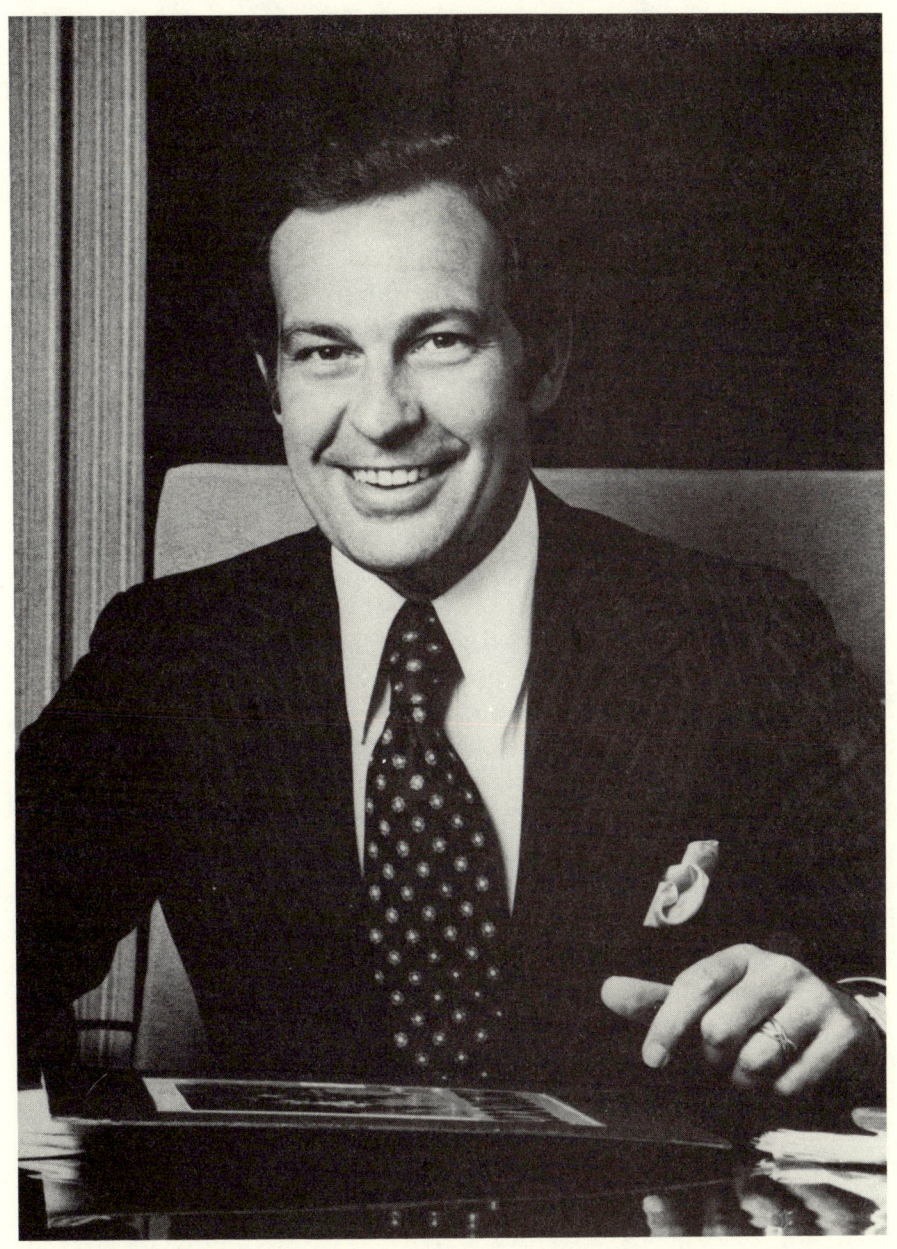

C. Carson Conrad

Born 1911

"Casey" Conrad has been executive director of the President's Council on Physical Fitness and Sports since 1970, having tuned up for the job by serving as a physical fitness consultant to Presidents Kennedy and Johnson. And Conrad looks so fit, so exuberantly healthy, that it's almost as though the federal government had gone to Central Casting for their man.

Although he exercised regularly from his boyhood through his college days (football, track, basketball), there was a time when he neglected training almost entirely.

"'I went into the soft life, only played golf, and ballooned up to two hundred fifteen pounds. I was a very happy, plump, and rather proficient golfer. Then I went for a checkup, and it turned out that that visit to the clinic was the beginning of a long, hard road back. Fortunately I had no organic problems, and my health was sound; I was one of the lucky ones. Since 1960 I've carried on a regular exercise program consisting of one hour of continuous, vigorous work each day.

"I took up tennis when I was fifty-eight years old," he continues. "I think you need to condition yourself for any sport, and you shouldn't depend on any one sport for your health.

"Many people don't realize what they could accomplish with a sensible regimen of exercise. You increase the metabolic rate to such an extent that after you've finished an hour of vigorous exercise, you still continue to burn the calories far and beyond the normal rate. That results in approximately a six-hundred-fifty-calorie expenditure in a one-hour workout."

An exercise regimen, he says, should give a man flexibility, muscular strength, and cardiorespiratory endurance. But, he adds, "Before a vigorous workout, a man should do about twenty minutes of stretching to ease his way into activity. The stretching movement has been growing the past four years. Some football teams have stretching coaches, it's gone that far."

Conrad begins his day lying on his back in bed. "I pull my knees up with my hands under my knees, and I try to bring them up to my chin; I pull them gradually tighter and hold that postion. I do thirty repetitions. Then I'm out of bed and do my stretching exercises."

At least once every day he works out with dumbbells and a barbell for muscular strength. He keeps a pair of twenty-five-pound dumbbells in his office and does twenty-five curls. In a gym he does bench presses with 125-pound barbells. Then it's onto a slant board, where for abdominal and back strength he does sit-ups with fingers laced behind his head. Conrad is convinced that a man who has no cardiovascular problems and is, say, "a young fifty can start weight lifting. Lifting weights in a horizontal position puts no strain on the spine."

Casey Conrad swims at least three times a week. He starts with Aqua Dynamics (bobbing) and then swims half a mile. (Bobbing is the reverse of an inverted surface dive. Conrad springs off the *bottom* of the pool and through leg-power thrust and arm pull he comes up out of the water to the waist, takes a deep breath, and then drops back to a squatting position and repeats.)

"The problem of many older men is lack of strength," he says. "And it's hard to stand straight without muscles to pull the shoulders back. Every man over forty-five should do stretching exercises morning and night plus sit-ups for his abdomen and back. Fitness is largely a matter of attitude; you've got to work at it. Put a little guts into your fitness program; listen to your body language."

According to Carson, the biggest problem his office has is convincing people that if they walk, breathe deeply, really *stride* out, they're exercising. "If I were king, I'd get out the whip and make people walk five miles a day. That would solve the majority of health problems today."

As for smoking: "I haven't smoked for years and years. You can't when you see the stuff that crosses my desk here. I believe somewhere between fifty and sixty-five percent of all premature deaths could be avoided with the right kind of exercise and the elimination of smoking. If a man has any kind of self-management about his life, he won't do it."

In 1960, Casey Conrad wrote the first paper on the benefits of jogging to be published in the United States, and he credits jogging with the fact that President Jimmy Carter despite the pressures of his job "has achieved a high level of physical conditioning and is in excellent health." In one year of his jogging two to five miles around the south lawn of the White House, Carter's weight has gone down from 157 to 148 pounds, and he has lowered his pulse rate from sixty beats per minute to forty beats per minute.

"It took some time for me to understand the difference between fitness for sport and fitness for living, which is getting conditioned for life," says Conrad. "It's not so much aging that takes its toll as it is the lack of work to maintain what you have." He hops up from behind his desk and picks up the pair of twenty-five-pound dumbbells. "I think if you wanted to kill me in a hurry, just sit me down and take away my incentive for activity."

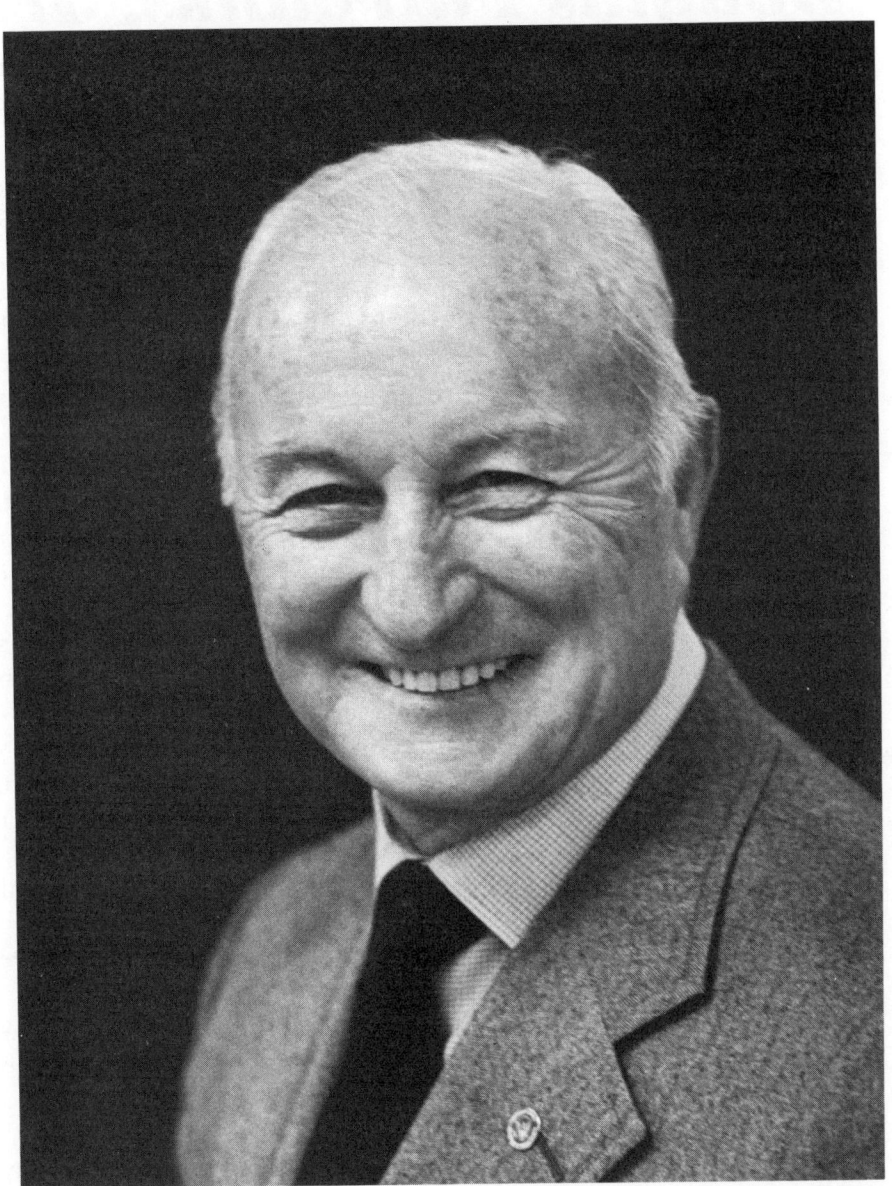

Douglas Fairbanks, Jr.

Born 1909

For my money, this is probably the world's best-dressed man. Whatever he puts on looks smart and grand, and no matter how well dressed you think you are, you somehow feel a trifle tacky compared to him. But it's certainly not any of his doing. Sitting behind his desk, wearing a gray single-breasted suit, a dove gray shirt with pale pink collar, striped tie, and a foulard silk pocket handkerchief, he seems almost embarrassed by his reputation as a modern-day Beau Brummell.

"Funnily enough, most of my clothes are old," he says. "This tie is twenty-five years old; this shirt was bought in Hong Kong ten years ago."

Of course, it's more than fine fabric and an extraordinary sense of color. "I saw him last week at dinner in New York," a fashion editor told me. "He was wearing a classic blue suit with white stripes and looked wonderful." We agreed that he was obviously born elegant.

He considers himself virtually retired as an actor. "I have my own film company, but I haven't made a movie in years. But once a year or once every eighteen months, I do a particular play under certain conditions: the right number of weeks; this particular director. It's rather like giving a concert after you've retired. I look upon it as a special event."

Active in business both here and abroad, he and his family have what he calls a second home. "I commute back and forth."

Fairbanks says his high-energy level "is constantly refreshed by an insatiable curiosity about life. I'm not the kind of person who has energy bursting out of my skin. It starts with the head and heart, and the energy comes up to meet it."

He has no particular exercise regimen. "I swim when I can, play tennis when I can, ski and water ski when I can, walk when I can, do what I can when I can. I watch my weight. My genes are lucky. I can play two or three sets of tennis, go horseback riding or fox hunting after a hiatus, and suffer no disturbances—at least so far. I just never get terrifically out of shape."

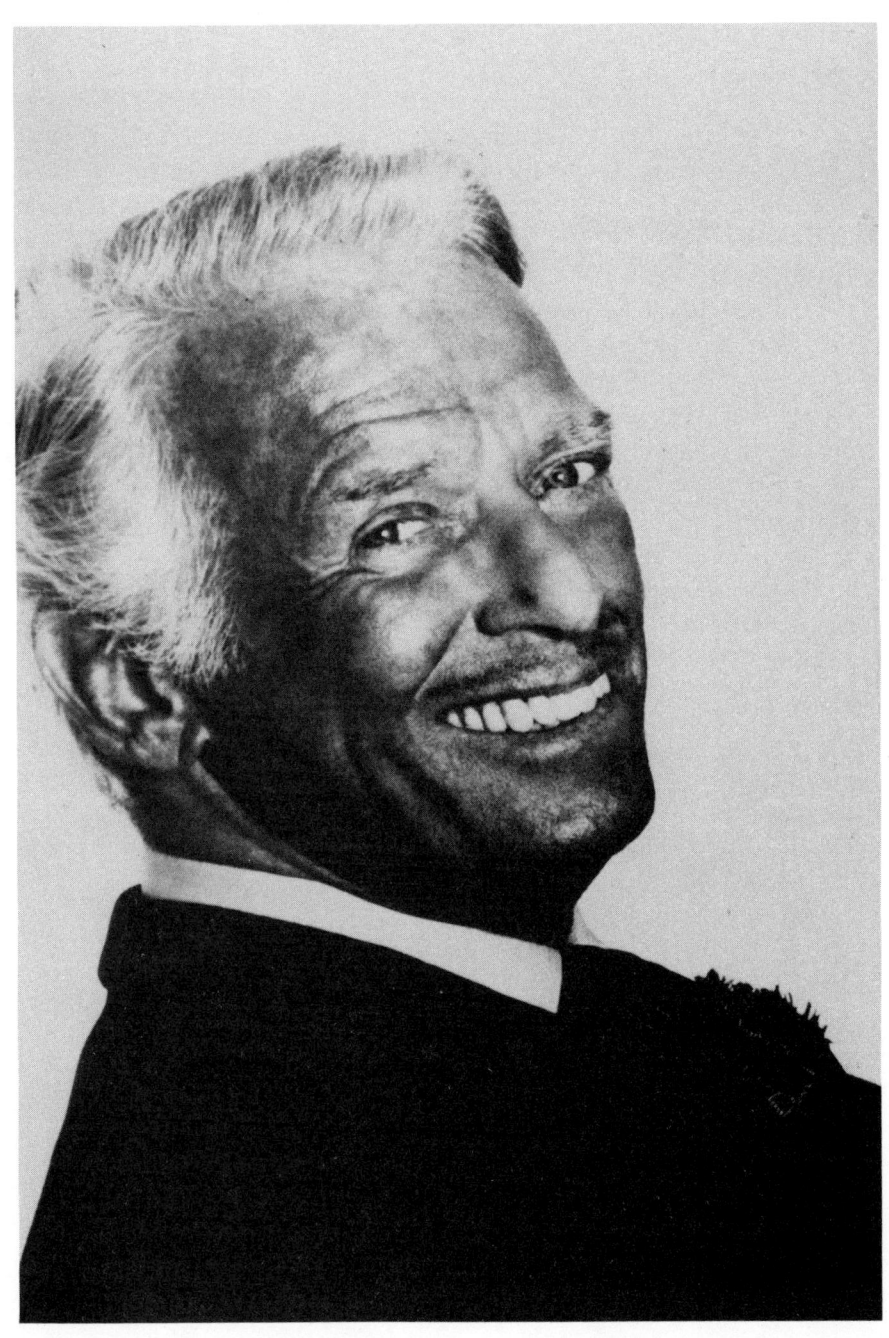

As far as diet goes: "My mother used to say that I'd eat stewed knitting if it was put in front of me. I listen to other people's theory on diet, try it a week or so, and go off it. The only time I really gained weight was when I gave up smoking altogether. I'd started getting a bronchial cough. I gained three or four pounds then."

His hair is gray—almost white—and he has a perpetual suntan. The effect is startling and cheerful. "Gray hair," he says, "runs in my mother's family. I started getting gray during the war—probably from fright. By forty I was nearly white. My mother was gray at twenty-six; my grandmother at eighteen. But my father didn't have one gray hair when he died, and he was fifty-six."

His world-famous father used to doodle the word "Success." "My father was very moody, but he didn't let it show. I am basically optimistic. I'm never in danger of ulcers, for I'm never too elated by good news, never too depressed by bad news, and I haven't been immune to either. I always reckon tomorrow's another day. I try to balance it off."

He has an autobiography in the making. It's just in the beginning stages, however. "Three people at this moment are doing a vast amount of research. The trouble is that I'm not much of an introvert."

William Fine

Born 1926

Bill Fine's thought on aging: "Work against it, and achieve a little bit of holding action." Just back from a few days in the sunshine of Palm Springs, California, he looks tanned, clear-eyed, and years younger than his calendar age, sitting in a red leather chair beneath a huge antique wall clock in his thirty-second-floor office. Fine obviously takes prime care of himself.

"I love the sun. I unclench my fists and feel all is right with the world. But I don't allow myself to burn; the first day in the sun I'm very, very cautious."

He hasn't smoked a cigarette in twenty years. He insists on getting seven hours' sleep. "Six makes me irritable. I never stay at a party past eleven. I try to see at least part of the eleven o'clock news every night; it's a ruse that keeps you from being fuzzy in the morning." He credits his extraordinary energy to a multiple vitamin from England called Pharmaton. "It's marvelous—has things in it that work in the aging process that our laws haven't passed yet." He buys it when he's traveling abroad.

Fine speaks in well-structured sentences that never fail to make a point—something you might expect from a man who was once publisher of a string of Hearst magazines and who is now president of Frances Denney, Inc., breathing new life into an aging cosmetic line via smart advertising and shrewd marketing.

Fine has a three-part recipe for staying youthful. One: Try to marry an athlete. "You're better off for it. Marry a woman who's a better skier than you are. Or one who plays a fantastic game of tennis so you don't have to hunt for a male partner." Two: Take minivacations. "I'll stop in the middle of the week, say, and go to a museum or a bookstore and look around. I come back mentally refreshed. If I find myself getting irritable, I'll stay home and work." Three: Have more than one career. "I find that one career makes you old. The age of specialization is a misfire. I sit on the boards of four other businesses."

Posture, he says, is something that the man approaching middle age had better learn fast. And he eschews long hair for any but the very young.

"We're going into an interesting period. Men really don't look as old as men did just a decade ago. There's much less variance with youth. There are more men now in the thirty-three to forty-four age-group. So if you're fiftyish, you're not comparing yourself to the twenty-year-olds, not copying their clothing."

Fine rides a bicycle weekends, pumping uphill because it's good for the legs. And there's a mountain behind the 150-year-old cottage he owns on six acres of land outside Galway, Ireland, which he makes it a point to climb as close to his birthday each year as possible.

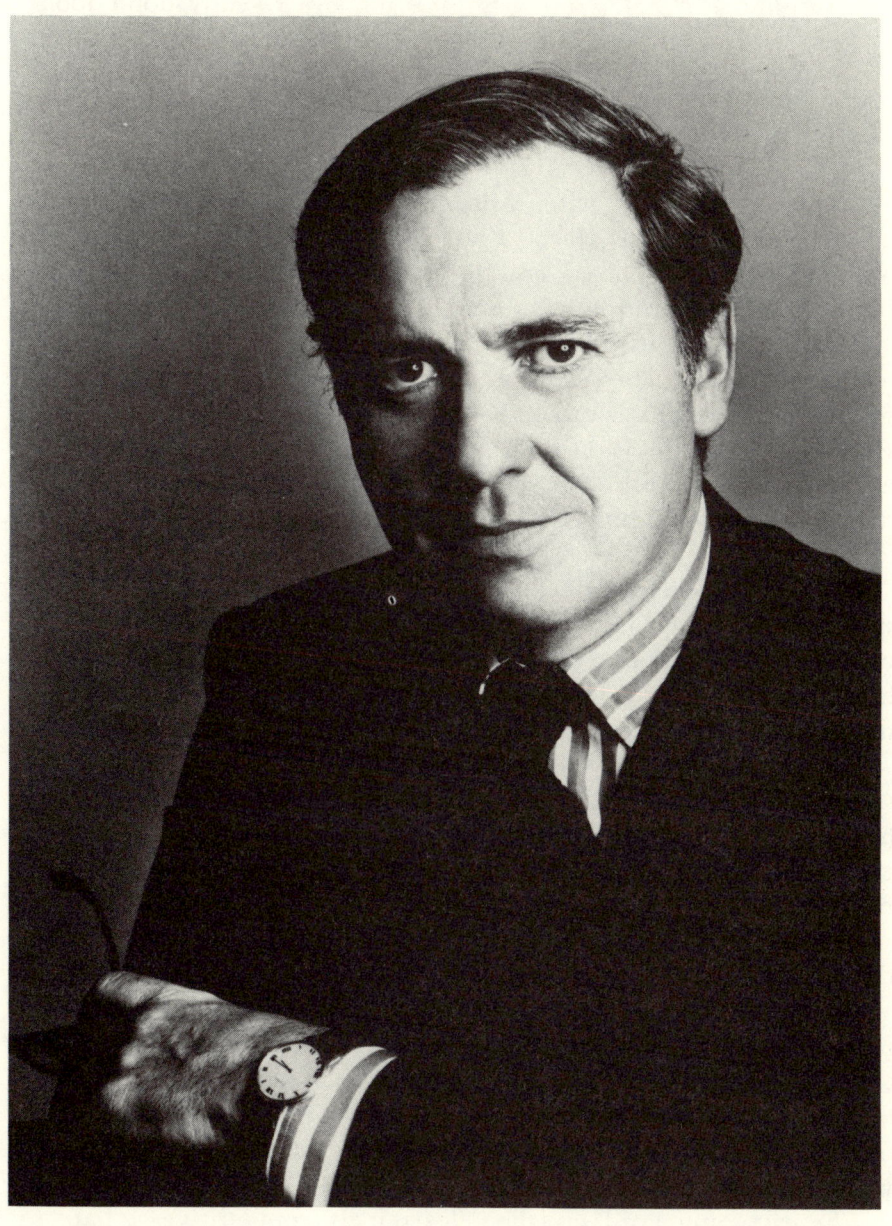

Gerard William Ford

Born 1924

Co-owner with his wife, Eileen, of Ford Models, the world's largest model agency, Jerry Ford weighs today exactly what he weighed when he played end for Notre Dame more than thirty years ago—205 pounds. But about fifteen years ago his weight ballooned to 235. He explains, "When you live in New York's business world, martini lunches are a way of life, and drinking is the worst problem for weight control. It's that extra thousand calories that kill you." These days Ford has cut down his business lunches to no more than one a week. "Most people I know have to be back in their offices in an hour. It's less chic to drink at lunch than it used to be."

He quit smoking in 1950. "I was fed up with smoker's hack and short wind and yellow fingers." He's also antisugar. "My mother was a later-day diabetic, and the doctor said as long as it's in your history. . . ." After a week of no sugar in his coffee, he found that not only didn't he miss it, but the very thought of it turned him off.

He and his wife travel abroad several times a year scouting for new models to bring back with them, and it's while traveling that he finds he has to practice self-discipline against the delicious food, especially the bread in France and Italy. "I have no sweet tooth, but I love good bread.

"The thing that impresses me most about my mature years is that the change in me isn't as great as I thought it would be thirty years ago. I can do everything I want to do, but less often, so I appreciate it even more than I used to when I play a tough game of squash—toe to toe with a guy ten years younger than I am—and I win. Then, of course, the bubble bursts—and happily—when a guy ten years older comes along and beats me. I'm just so impressed with people who keep physically active all their lives."

The easygoing Ford says he's "extremely competitive. I hate to come in second, but I don't think you have to be highly nervous to be competitive."

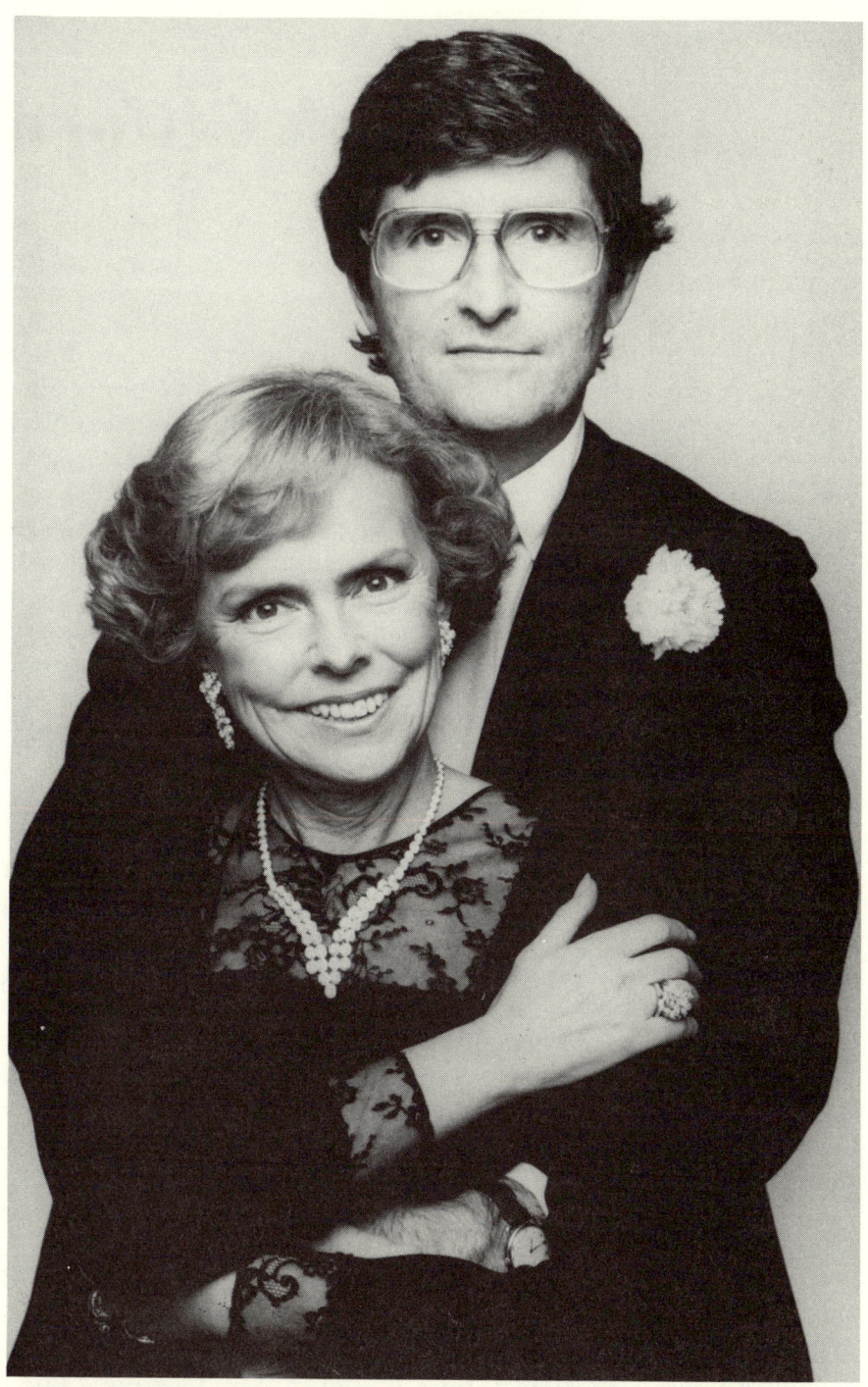

Gerard and Eileen Ford. PHOTO BY JAMES MOORE.

Frank Gifford

Born 1930

That an ex-athlete invariably turns to fat is, according to Frank Gifford, "a gross cliché." He weighs 190, the same as he weighed during the twelve years he played football with the New York Giants, when he set Giant records that still stand, including most touchdowns (78) and most yards gained pass receiving (5,484).

Togged out in jeans, boots, and an open-necked shirt with sleeves rolled to the elbows, he's just returned from two days spent rafting on a river in Maine. He's sitting in his office at ABC-TV, where he works as a sports commentator, and along with the tennis and ski trophies is the Emmy he was awarded for the 1976–77 season as television's Outstanding Sports Personality. But except for the pair of telephones on his desk that ring almost incessantly, there's little about him that suggests a frenetic schedule.

"I do nothing with any great intensity—good or bad," he says. "Basically I don't do anything in excess, including exercise. I stay physically active, but nothing on a routine basis. I do a little bit of everything—tennis, golf, ski. I swim mostly to cool off. My wife, on the other hand, runs ten miles almost every day; she plays tournament tennis and teaches aerobic dancing. When I feel I'm getting soft in the gut, I do sit-ups. I know what certain exercises will do for certain muscles, but actually I'm a better teacher than a practitioner.

"I walk a lot—and fast—to get someplace; I enjoy it. I don't pay much attention to diet. I'm not a huge eater, but I eat everything. I drink a lot of milk because it tastes good. It's sort of like having a thermometer in my head. I know what my body needs—not what is a protein, what is a starch."

Gifford smokes two packs of cigarettes a day. "I enjoy it. Of course, I realize it's not good for me, but I enjoy it. Still, I'm the first to tell my kids not to smoke."

Gifford is also a spokesman for a line of suits and a wine. "But I drink nothing, not even wine, during the daytime. I know that it

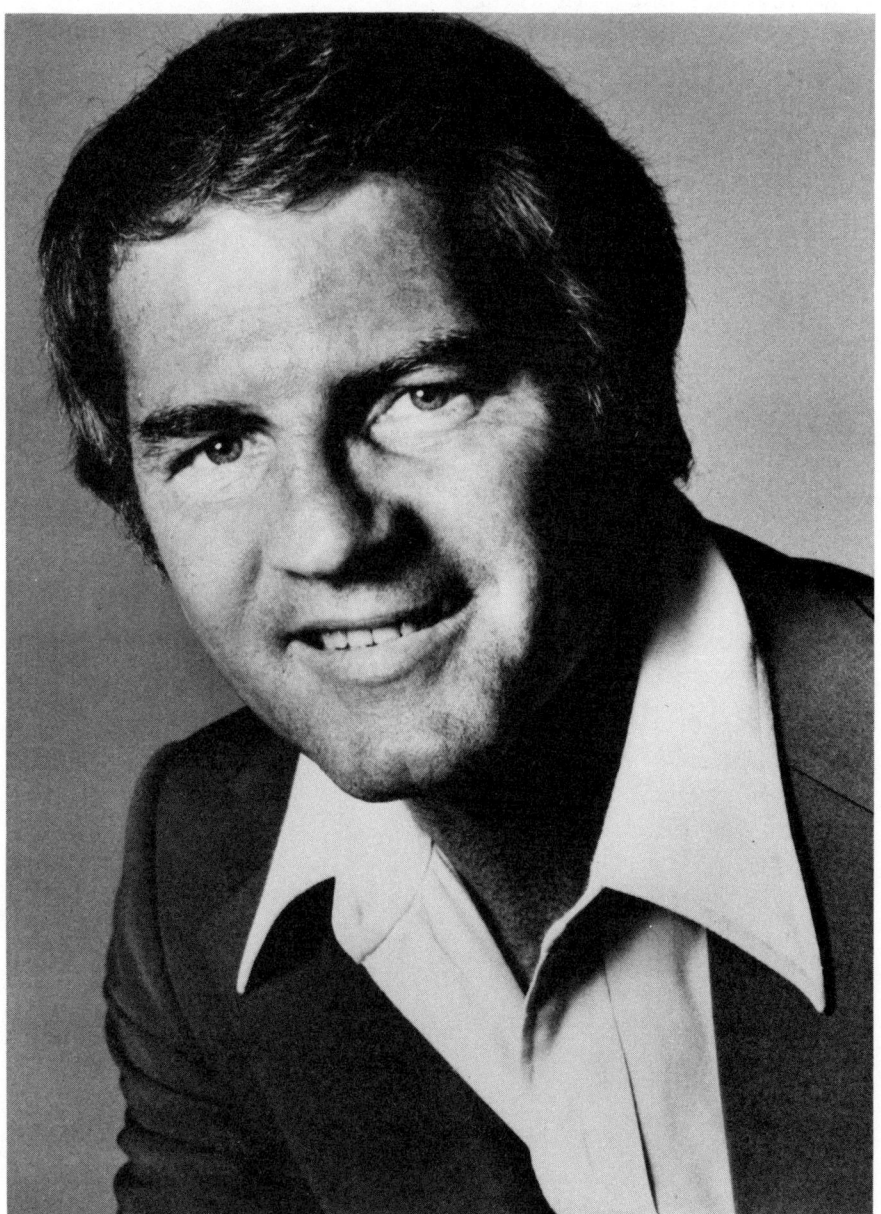
PHOTO BY GARY BERNSTEIN.

would hurt my performance before the camera. I've seen too many tragedies come out of drinking."

He played his final season of football in 1964, the year he was named Sportsman of the Year. Today, at the half-century mark, looking about thirty-five, he says, "I can do everything I once did, but I can't do it as hard or as long."

Mark Hatfield

Born 1922

The outer office of the senator from Oregon is full of Portland memorabilia. Notable is a huge photograph of "Portland's Great Flood, June, 1894," showing men in bowler hats either sitting in rowboats or standing in water outside a department store. In Hatfield's private office it's Lincoln memorabilia, and there is a Lincolnesque quality about the man himself.

Mention stress, and he knocks on the wood of his antique desk. "So far I've avoided manifestations of stress. I believe you can reduce stress by taking certain vitamins, but even before this, I discovered the secret of avoiding stress. You must have a well-defined philosophy of life, not just for the moment but forever and eternity. Then you can keep a perspective on the importance of events. You have to have this perspective of things in a time frame, both backwards and forwards. Ask yourself how vitally important an issue was, say, ten years ago and where is it today. Look to the future. Time is eternity. Too many people are too busy to develop a philosophy; a philosophy is the heart and soul of life.

"Back home in Oregon I'll stand a hundred feet on a bank above the ocean and watch the tide and the waves beating against the rocks, and this also gives me a perspective of self, of ego.

"Also, I've learned how to relax, to float out from my mind and spirit those things that can become barnacles and fossils. I don't take a briefcase home with me at the end of the day. If work isn't finished, too bad. What if I'd gotten ill? Somebody else would have to take care of it.

"One needs a change of pace, a change of issues, of views. And lastly, try to have a diversity of friendships. I don't constantly talk politics. Some of my colleagues fraternize only with colleagues. I enjoy my colleagues, but not night after night after night. To get down to the end of the road, to retirement, and what's left? To see the end of your career and to be lost. People like that are lonely, disillusioned. It's very dangerous to get so specialized. There are other fields I could go into and enjoy—the academic community, for example."

Hatfield became intensely interested in nutrition while serving on the Food and Nutrition Committee. "By way of the different people I met then, I began to read about vitamins, minerals, and food supplements. Now I take copious quantities of vitamin C; it accelerates the healing process—both my dentist and surgeon have commented on how fast I heal. I also take B complex, E, A, and D, zinc, calcium, potassium, niacin, lecithin. I'm my own doctor. Doctors have very little training in nutrition, but now I see a growing awareness. I think the public is often ahead, politically and medically."

He gave up smoking on April 15, 1954. "I remember the date very well." He consumes no hard liquor. "It's a drug." And he does calisthenics for fifteen minutes, in the morning and again in the evening: sit-ups, push-ups, knee bends, and side twists. "But I enjoy swimming and hiking more than anything else."

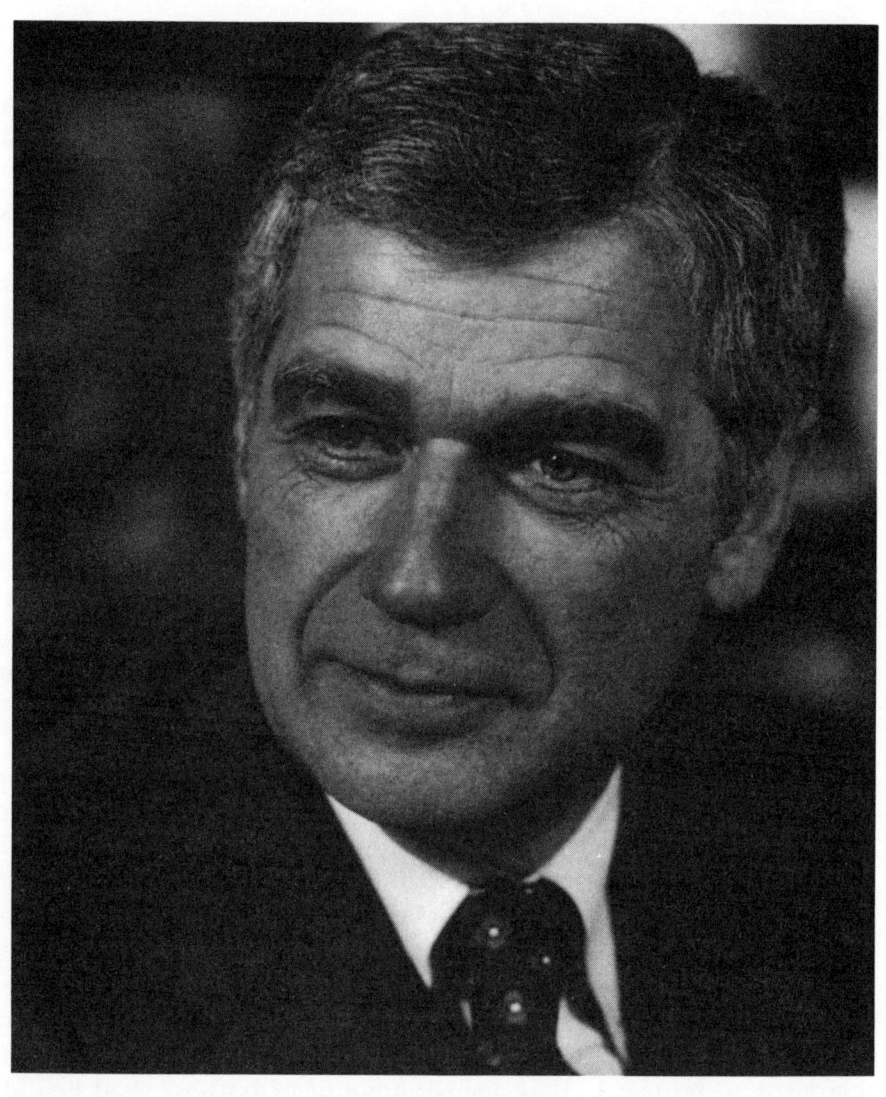

Gayelord Hauser
Born 1894

Gayelord Hauser has been called the Father of Modern Nutrition. That's the inscription at the base of a six-foot statue of him standing now in the newly named Hauser Square in Kyoto, Japan. The day I met him, he had just gotten back from there and, even more recently, from a one-hour three-mile walk around the reservoir in New York's Central Park. "I walk one hour a day, every day—fast, nonstop. It's a heart massage."

The following day he'd be off to lecture in Boston, and after that he'd appear at a nutritionists' convention in Brussels. Home is a six-acre estate on the shore of Sicily, but he's rarely there. He's constantly on the go. He certainly must be weary of hearing that he is his own best advertisement for what he preaches: natural foods and all-around natural living. Still, he takes it in stride, as he apparently does everything else. Six feet three inches tall and erect as a military officer, suntanned, with a head full of hair, a mouth full of his own teeth, and the same weight (185 pounds) he was when he wrote his first best-seller, *Look Younger, Live Longer*, more than thirty years ago, Gayelord Hauser is a phenomenal man.

"I'm an optimist," he announces. Very much, he says, like the Russians in the province of Georgia who live well over a hundred years. "They're optimists, too, nature lovers, eating honey and black bread and breathing in that good mountain air."

He's bombarded with questions after every lecture. He tells people, "It's not a matter of what you like but what your body needs. As you get older, eat less." He's against milk—"Nondairy countries don't have arthritis"—and uses only skim milk and yogurt. "Yogurt is fermented." He's against margarine. "It's unnatural, more dangerous than butter; I allow a small amount of butter." And he's all for walking. "As the Russians say, 'Movement is life. Sitting is death.' Maintain a steady, comfortable pace, and don't stop. Take long, long steps. You may start out tired, but you'll end up refreshed. Why? Because you're pumping so much oxygen. A low-calorie diet plus daily walking equals the world's biggest lifesaver." He's also

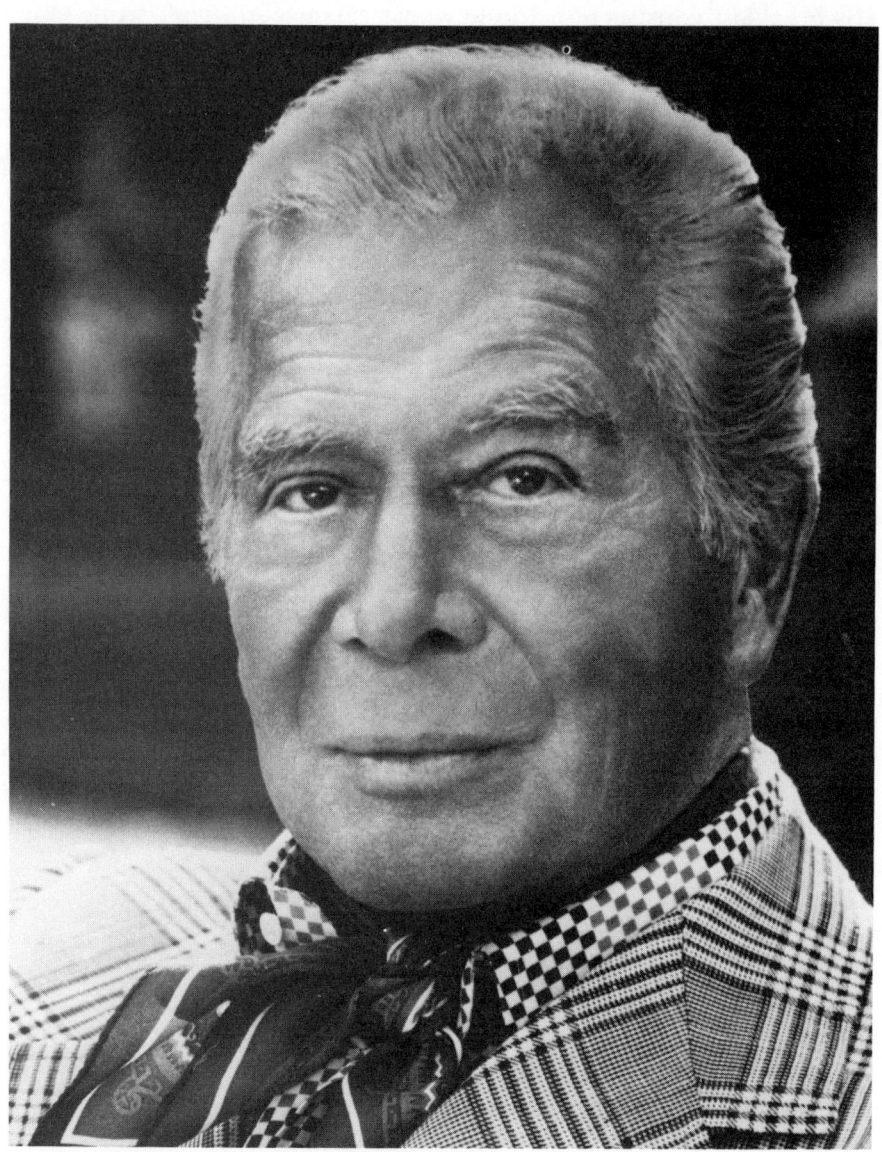

enthusiastic about vitamin C. "It's wonders are never-ending."

Hauser would like to lose five pounds. "The less I weigh, the better for my heart," he says, while patting his washboard-flat stomach. His breakfast consists of a whole wheat cereal with fresh fruit. Once a day he drinks *café au lait,* and after that it's tea or herb tea. He has eggs no more than two or three times a week. "Soft-boiled, and I spike them with powdered onion or powdered garlic or herbs, rather than salt and pepper. The more herbs you digest, the less fat you need." He drinks a quart of water each day, and this, too, he spikes "with fresh lemon." He advises his followers to start luncheon and dinner with a salad. "It takes the big hunger away." And he always has fresh fruit for dessert.

When visiting the USSR recently, he met with the minister of nutrition. He says that Russian soldiers carry sacks over their shoulders containing wheat kernels, onion, garlic. "Our boys eat Hershey bars," says Hauser sadly, adding, "I am more afraid of Russian vitality than the bomb."

He'd like to establish what he calls a VIP Farm for Men, where they would be taught in two weeks how to eat properly. "Men are more faithful to good nutrition than women who too often are on a carousel diet." Meantime, he's completing a new cookbook titled *Tender, Loving Cooking.* "I find that people who care are good cooks; they cook with their eyes, ears, and hearts."

Always looking to the future, he has plans to start his autobiography. He figures that at ninety he may take time off, go home to Sicily, sit down, and work on it. He doesn't require eyeglasses to read now, and he doesn't expect he'll need them then either.

Jim Jensen

Born 1926

Jim Jensen, CBS-TV anchorman, does more than simply read the news with resonant voice and flawless diction to 18 million viewers; he's a working journalist. He goes out and covers the news, then comes back and writes it. Rushing to a fire in 1966, he suffered an automobile accident that necessitated a spinal fusion. After a long hospitalization he was wearing a back brace and walking with a cane. "I decided at the time that I would never be like that again. I asked my doctor what I should do. His answer was exercise. I was on skis one month later."

Nowadays Jensen skis, swims, snorkels, and works out at a YMCA near the television studio five days a week for one continuous hour; he runs, stretches, lifts weights, and does calisthenics. "My workouts at the Y are probably vanity," he says, "my wanting to look as good as I can for as long as I can. I'll sometimes go roaring on by past an old gent with a cane. That will be me one day, and I know I won't like it—but it's inevitable."

Jensen also pitches on the CBS softball team. The team plays about eighty games a year in the course of which it raises some $100,000 for charity. "Playing ball is probably protracted adolescence, but I enjoy the total escape the game offers. Everything's black and white. There are so many gray areas in life, but there's never any question about which team won. It's the total simplicity I like. In baseball there are a lot of absolutes."

Jensen weighs a rangy 195 pounds. There's not an ounce of surplus flesh on his six-foot-four-inch frame. When he was in his teens and early twenties, he was skinny and self-conscious about his appearance. He appears proud of the way he looks now as he walks around the newsroom in his shirt sleeves—a media superstar with a six-figure annual income. "I can be a damn pain in the ass," he says, "but I'm a lot more tolerant than I used to be. No longer so damnably narcissistic. I hope I'm wiser, too, more at peace with myself than I was in my thirties.

"I have tremendous stamina. I worked last night here at CBS

until five in the morning writing. I made a speech today at noon, then did two telecasts, and between them went to the Y to exercise. Right now I'm doing a whole series on energy. I spent a day in a coal mine; there's another segment on nuclear energy, and that's very complicated. You have to study constantly in this job; you never have enough background. Luckily I can get by with four hours' sleep. I guess I have a different kind of clock in me." When he feels the need for more energy, he sends out for a peanut butter and honey sandwich or a candy bar.

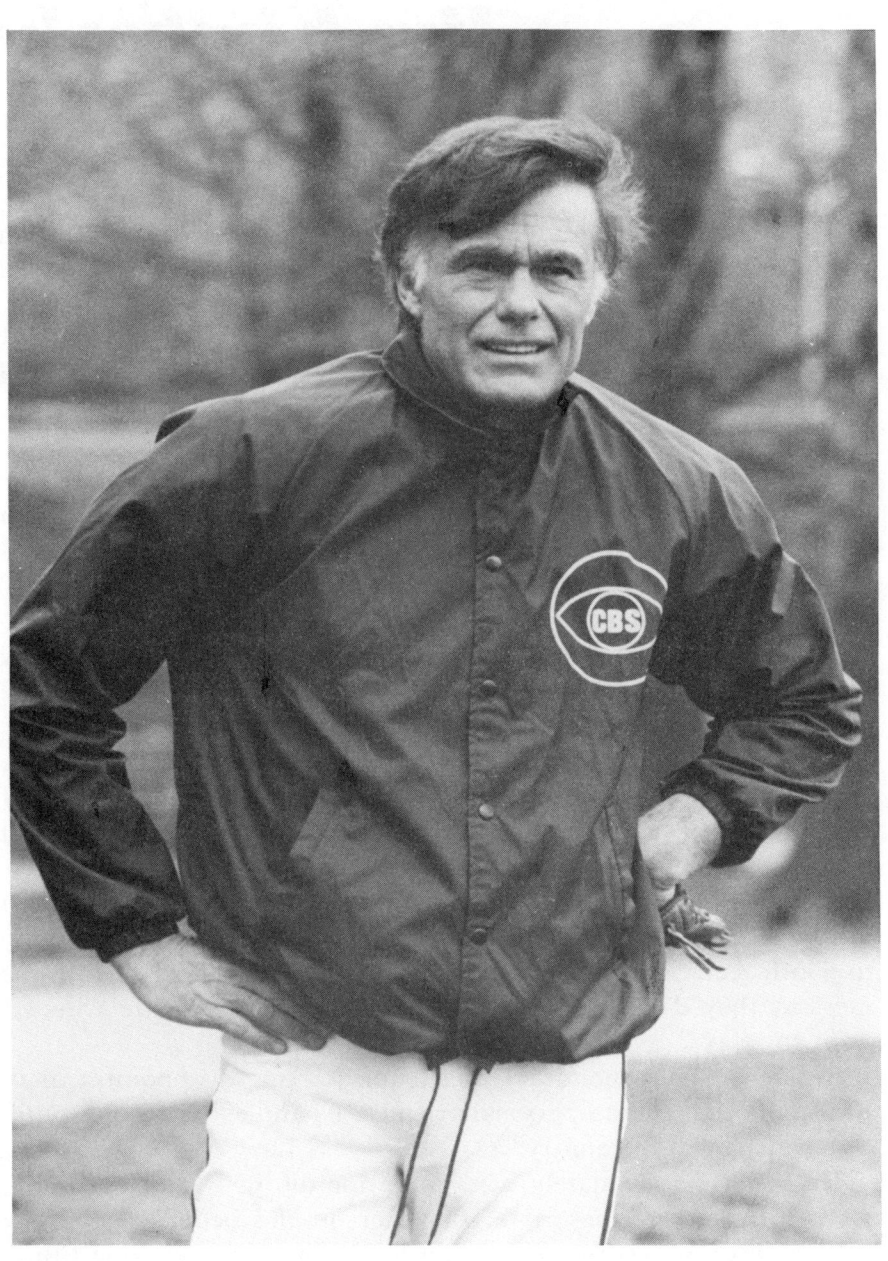

Jim Kimberly
Born 1907

The grandson of the founder of the Kimberly-Clark Corporation was carrying a lot of gold on him the day we met: gold tie clasp; gold belt buckle; gold watch with gold band; gold cuff links; and, most arresting, a gold earring in his right ear. "It's a personal thing," he explains. "Goes back to World War Two. A group of us formed a little club. There were six to start; now there are only two of us alive. . . ."

Kimberly, white-haired and deeply tanned, comes from a long-lived line. The next day he and his wife were going to visit with his ninety-nine-year-old aunt in California. His father died at ninety-one; his father's sister, at a hundred and one.

He retired from Kimberly-Clark at fifty-six, but he doesn't consider himself to be retired in the full sense of that word, for now he's the Florida commissioner of the Port of Palm Beach, an elective office. There were 53,000 votes cast, and he won by 48. Campaigning, he says, he discovered that "it takes a lot of stamina, a lot of drive to convince people you can do a better job than your opponent, and furthermore, you've got to *prove* it later. I've found any political promise you make, you've got to keep or else."

His legal residence is in Palm Beach, where he first went in 1925 to visit a college roommate. He enjoys the climate and the proximity to South America. "I've given up on cities. They used to intrigue me, but they don't anymore. I've reached a time of life where I want to relax."

Kimberly is also honorary consul for Jordan by appointment of King Hussein, a close personal friend. "I handle the whole southeastern part of the country."

He believes passionately in exercise for the body and the brain, too, which he describes as "a computer beyond belief."

"You have to exercise your brain by reading, by reviewing things that are important for you to know. Read *The Decline and Fall of the Roman Empire*, and there you'll find almost a direct parallel to what we're going through today. I don't know the man who can step

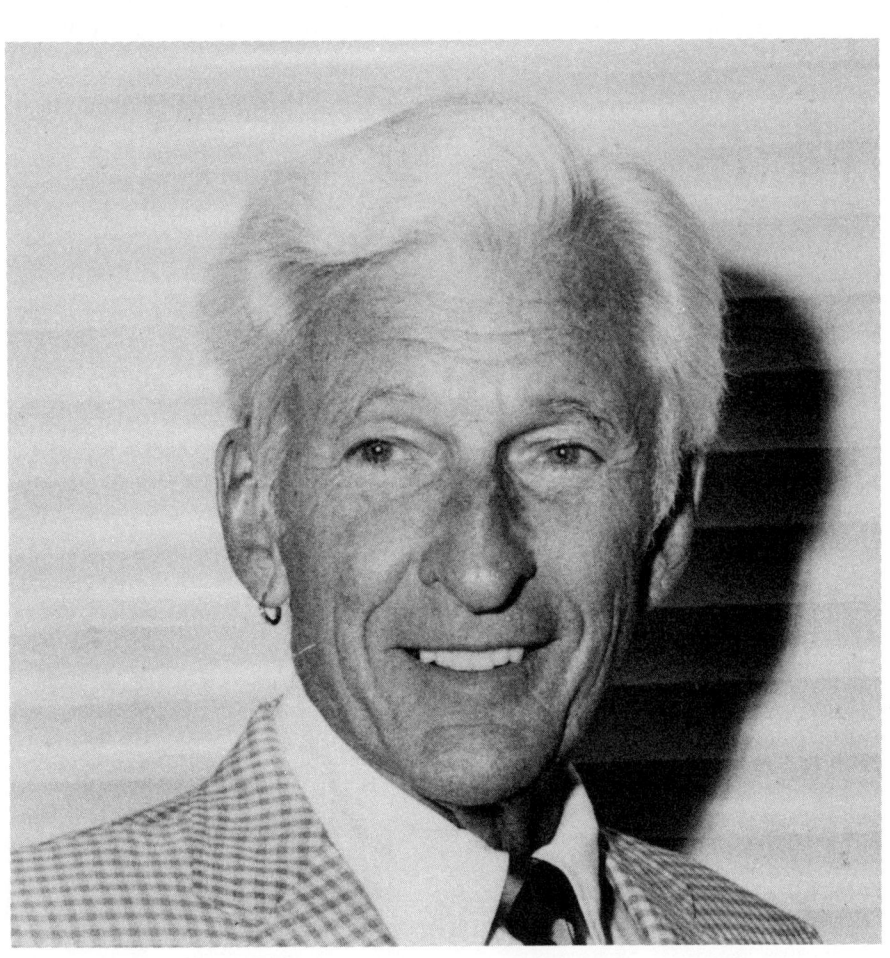

in and change things around. We have no confidence, no faith in any of them, and when you don't have confidence in your leaders, you lose faith in the whole system."

Six feet tall, Kimberly at 157 pounds is only seven pounds heavier than when he was on the crew at MIT. "It's a very demanding sport; most people don't realize that. What training it takes! The top crew at Henley last year was Yugoslavian, and what athletes they were!" Right now his sports are deep-sea fishing and auto racing. "And I do a lot of swimming. I have a pool and swim every day. I keep the water quite warm—in the high eighties. I swim and exercise in the water, too. It's buoyant and doesn't put a strain on your body. When you're young, I believe in more violent exercise. I like violent sports; violence when it's well done is interesting. But after a certain period in life everything should be done in moderation. Do enough exercise to keep the muscles toned up.

"My normal sleep cycle is five hours. Some men at my age take naps, but God, I never have time for that! Every day there are things to accomplish."

Bill Loock

Born 1920

You probably grew up seeing Bill Loock in glossy ads for the kinds of suits you couldn't afford to buy—yet. As male models go, he's a phenomenon. He started his career in 1945 and hasn't stopped modeling since, although long ago he started an insurance brokerage office on the side. In the intervening thirty-five years his appearance has scarcely changed, except that today he weighs five pounds less than when he played football at Chapel Hill. The aristocratic Edwardian looks are still handsomely intact, and his thick dark brown hair is only lightly flecked with gray.

"Of course, I'm very conscious of how I look," he says. "I'm in a business where people praise you all your life. I'm vain, but I hope without being a pain in the ass."

Loock has a hunch that his good looks and good health are hereditary. "My father was a very young-looking man all his life until he had a stroke at sixty-five, and then he aged overnight. I was modeling with young girls until I was fifty-four. I felt kind of ridiculous about it; I had a daughter their age. I don't fool anybody about my age. I don't pretend to be younger than I am, and I'm not totally convinced that men my age want to see men my age in ads."

Admittedly he had no particular regard for his health until he was fifty. "There's nothing worse than getting older and feeling lousy." He gave up smoking then. Now he drinks white wine at cocktail parties. "You're kidding yourself on wine really. It's no better or worse than a martini for your liver. But I find going to cocktail parties, people resent it if you don't drink something."

Loock has always been athletic: tennis; squash; golf. On the golf course he wears one of his all-time favorite hats: a large-brimmed plantation straw sporting a band of pheasant feathers. And he has a swimming pool at home in Connecticut.

Growing older, he finds that he doesn't have as much desire to eat. Still, he watches the amounts he consumes. "Let's face it; otherwise, you can't expect not to gain weight."

He confesses that he spent too much time in the sun in his youth.

His good skin managed to survive because it's oily. "Sun is very bad for your skin as you age. I was recently in Palm Beach, and there at high noon, women forty and fifty were lapping it up. It's just got to destroy their skin."

Doesn't a man with hair like his and skin like his have any maintenance tips to pass on? Well, he shaves with a regular razor and doesn't use an after-shave. As for shampoo, "I use anything that happens to be in the bathroom."

FORD MEN Plaza 3-6500
              688-8627 TV

BILL LOOCK

SIZE	40R
HEIGHT	6'1"
WAIST	33
INSEAM	32
SHIRT	15½-34
HAIR	Brown
EYES	Brown
SHOE	10½C
HAT	7¼
GLOVE	9½

SAG   A.F.T.R.A.

EXCELLENT HANDS

David Mahoney

Born 1923

I first became aware of David Joseph Mahoney back in the 1940s, when Robert Ruark, a noted author and widely syndicated newspaper columnist, devoted an entire column to the twenty-five-year-old whiz kid who was making $500 per week in a Madison Avenue advertising agency. That was roughly like $1,000 per week today, and since I was making something like $60 per week at the time, I was mightily impressed. Three years later he opened his own agency. I might have forgotten all about Mahoney, however, except that he made it impossible to do so. His career quickly became legendary: president of the Good Humor ice cream company at thirty-three; next stop, number two man at Colgate-Palmolive.

In 1979 *The New York Times* duly reported that there were twelve industrial executives whose incomes had exceeded $1 million the previous year. Number one on the list was David Joseph Mahoney, chairman of Norton Simon, Inc.

> Mr. Mahoney, 55 years old, received $1,196,667 in salary and bonus last year, up from $800,000 in 1977. But company proxy statements show that gains from stock options and stock appreciation rights added $1,120,388 to his total income from the conglomerate, which makes and markets goods in the fields of food, cosmetic and fashions, among others. . . .

His beige, brown, and white office on the forty-sixth floor of a Park Avenue skyscraper has, along with fine Oriental antiques, a sofa pillow that reads, "Bless the Bureaucracy." Mahoney himself has the kind of energy that seems to run rampant around the room. He credits it to "The joy of living. I enjoy this world," he says. "Excitement creates its own energy. Depression robs energy." It's difficult to imagine him ever being really depressed.

A European business writer who interviewed Mahoney recently noted: "The chain-smoking, coffee-quaffing boss of Norton Simon has the looks and skills to attract attention everywhere." And so he has. He's acknowledged to be directly responsible for Norton Simon,

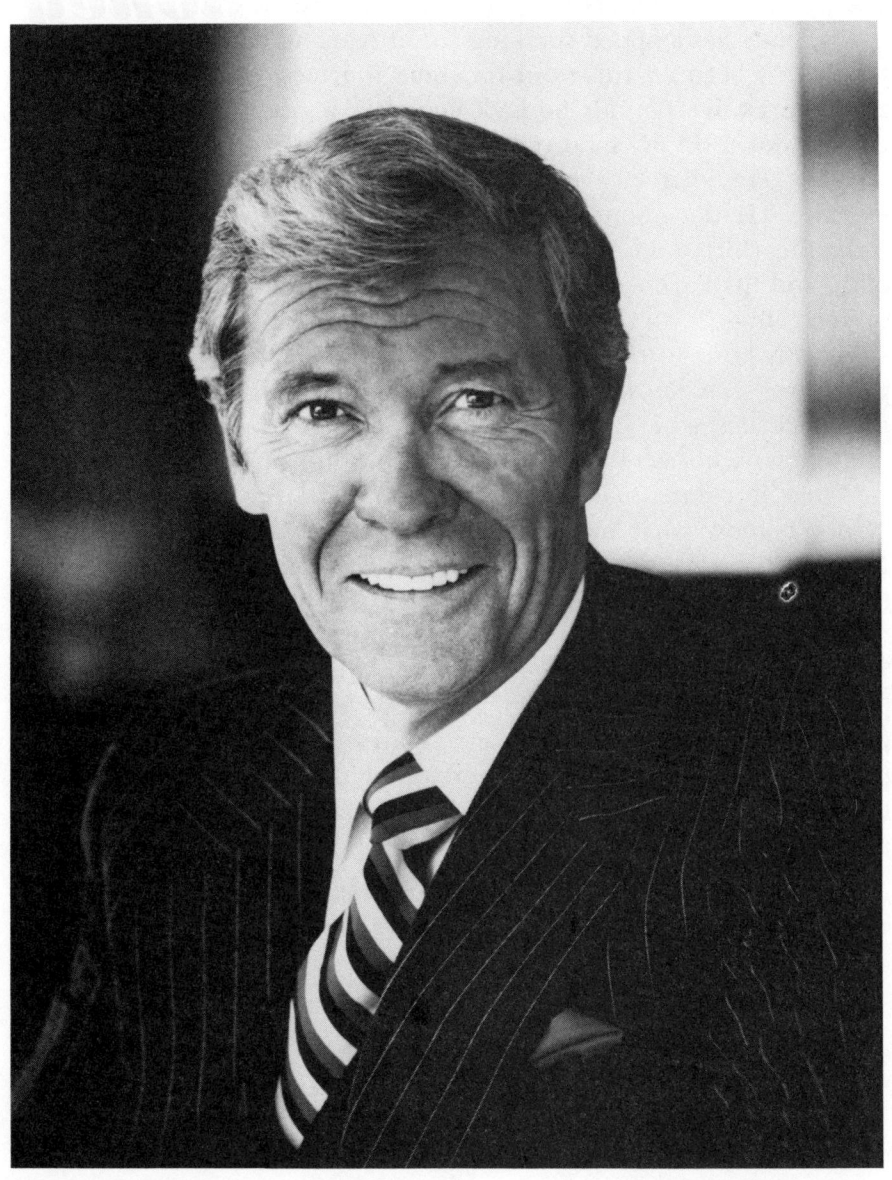

Inc.'s success story—one that includes the operation of ten corporations, among them Avis, Inc., Canada Dry, Max Factor, Hunt-Wesson Foods, Glass Containers Corporation, and United Can.

Mahoney has stopped smoking—or at least he had when I last saw him. He'd been off the weed for some fourteen weeks and had just shed the twelve pounds he had gained as a result. "I got it off by cutting down on my food intake; that's the only way I know to lose weight." He doesn't have as much time as he would like for regular exercise. He plays squash and tennis "when I can," and he tries to walk the thirty-odd blocks that stretch between his Park Avenue office and his Park Avenue apartment. He credits his fitness "mostly to good stock."

He was born in the Bronx, son of an Irish crane operator, and a priest who has known him since boyhood recalls: "He would say that he'd succeed and make a lot of money. He'd say that flatly, and the fellows who were playing stickball would laugh at him."

When it comes to analyzing his motivations, Mahoney admits, "I don't know what makes me tick, to be really honest about it." Money? "Less so then it was. Money alone won't make you happy, money alone won't make you secure, but it is a part of it."

Rumor has it that he is mulling over a run for the White House. Several of the books on the shelves in his office have to do with politics, *The New Language of Politics*, for one. But speaking of his plans for when his NSI contract expires in 1985, he says, "I will probably end up running a major foundation in the United States, involved in education and science, and taking care of what I think are social needs."

Either way you'll be hearing about this handsome, hard-charging gamesman for a long time to come.

Charles Percy

Born 1919

"Chuck" Percy's seniority in the United States Senate entitles him to an office on a lower floor of the Dirksen Building, but the senator from Illinois chooses to remain on the fourth floor so that every time there's a vote he can walk the stairs. The day I visited with him, he'd been up since 5:00 A.M. but looked as though he'd just gotten back from a long vacation.

"I always enjoy life," he says. "Every day is a great challenge, full of satisfaction. Campaigning is mentally taxing, physically exhausting, but when you like what you're doing—well, you find the energy."

Percy tries to get a good workout in the Senate gym at least twice a week: rides a stationary bike; skips rope; does push-ups. "The Senate gym was, I believe, put there when it was found that statistically congressmen had such a high mortality rate. So little time for exercise, and weekends they go back home and spend their time visiting their constituents."

Percy makes time for regular exercise. "I play tennis a couple of times a week, and I always travel with a swimsuit and a skip rope in my luggage. I try to stay where there's a pool. That's why I'm addicted to Holiday Inns; all of them have a pool. I do at least forty skips with a rope, starting with skip walking and go on to a double jump."

He has a trim, compact physique; he doesn't count calories. "I simply eat sensibly. Taste is an acquired thing. People get used to sweets. Children start their day with frosted cereals and become addicted to sweetening. Years ago I gave up sugar in tea and coffee; I find they taste just as good without it. I have a normal sugar intake; most Americans consume twice as much sugar as they need. I stay away from deep-fried foods. I take whole-grain cereals and skim milk. I have a good appetite. I certainly don't starve myself, but I burn up the calories."

Like many of the men I interviewed, Percy is an inveterate walker. "Mrs. Percy and I walk a lot; we've found that our home in Georgetown offers us a variety of walks. And we like to bike along the canal. I also did a lot of skiing when I was in business; I had more free time then and could get away more. Now I ski on an occasional three-day weekend and take ten days at Christmas and go to Vail or Aspen. I met my wife at a ski resort."

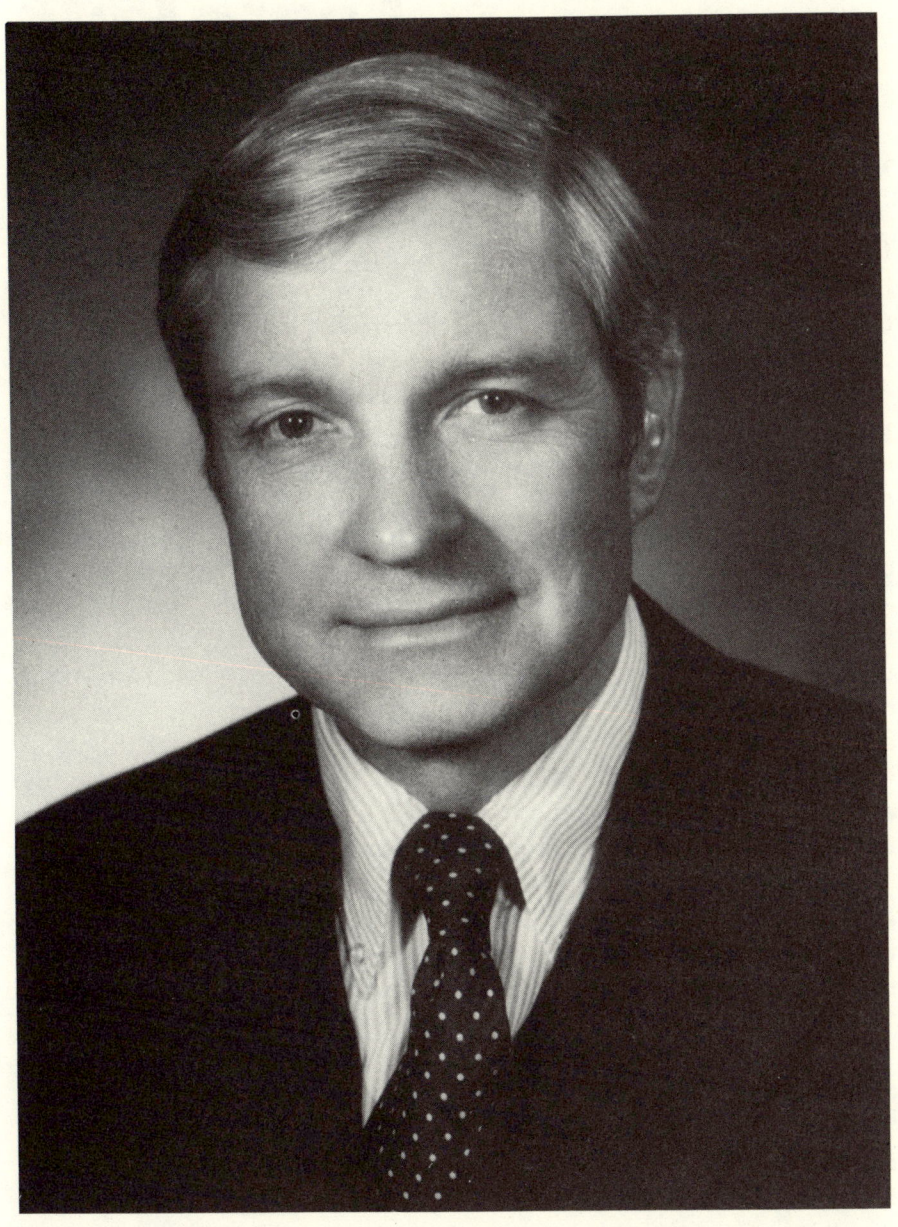

Louis Polk

Born 1930

"Bo" Polk, with a string of venture-capital successes to his credit, is chairman and chief executive of Leisure Dynamics, Inc., a game, hobby, and publishing company and leader in the development of electronic games. His New York apartment has a splendid river view and looks as though it might have been designed as a backdrop for a film about a jet age tycoon. And why not? Polk was once president of Metro-Goldwyn-Mayer. Marshall McLuhan looked around the premises one evening and decided, "It would be a difficult place to be depressed."

Polk weighs the same today as he did when he was captain of an undefeated football team at Phillips Andover Academy. He works at staying fit. "I pay attention to how my body feels," he says. He plays tennis, skis, sails, swims, scuba dives, and jogs—and takes a sauna twice a week. "I'll always find time to run if I'm not getting any exercise at all. After all, you can run anywhere, anytime." At the start of the ski season he works out with weights to strengthen his legs. About the only sport he doesn't participate in is golf. "On a tennis court you get three times the exercise in less than half the time." He has no idea where his golf clubs are nowadays.

He doesn't smoke, he eats sensibly, and he avoids hard liquor. Breakfast is two glasses of freshly squeezed orange juice, and he never takes coffee. Lunch is usually soup and salad, while dinner may be fowl and steamed vegetables. But so far as dessert is concerned, "I'm very carefree about that."

He walks crosstown to his office every morning, where he tries to transfer the discipline he's learned from sports to his business life. "I tend not to let things get me down. You know you can win no matter how far you're behind." Athletic, team-oriented men, he finds, come into business with a real desire to compete. "They have the drive that a lot of other men haven't learned to deal with. On an athletic team you learn how to relax while in a tremendously stressful situation. In business there's a lot of intensity, but it's self-serving. Personally I make a big difference between *positive-* and

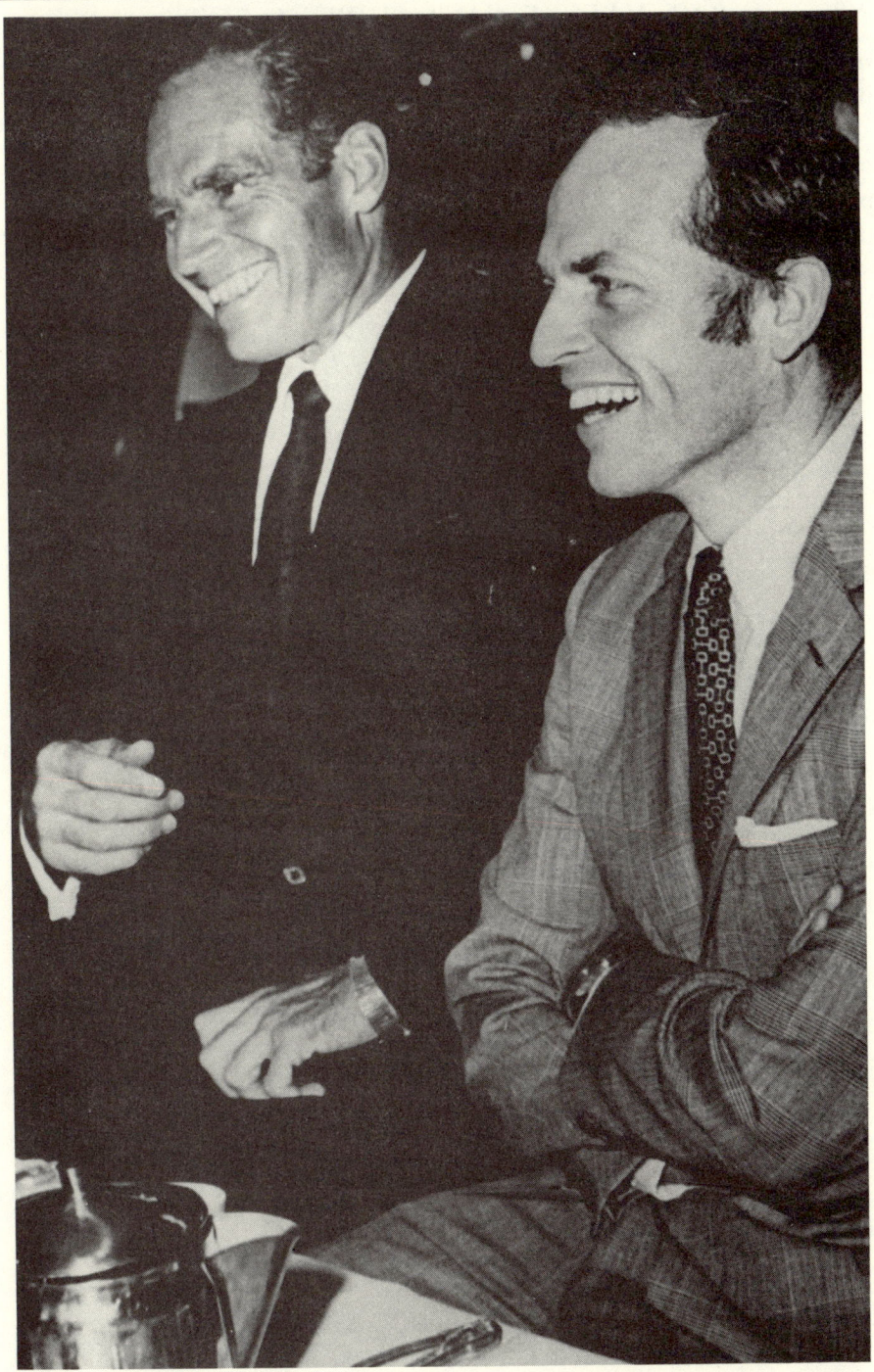
"Bo" Polk and his friend and tennis partner, Charlton Heston.

negative-type energy, genuine enthusiasm versus merely being overly intense."

Last year he climbed Mount Kenya with his eighteen-year-old son. "In the early stages of adjustment he was a little bit of a complainer, but the last two days all I saw was his tail end. It was then that I realized the difference in what it means to be eighteen and forty-nine!"

Bobby Short
Born 1924

"I have to worry about myself like a prizefighter would," says singer-pianist Bobby Short, one of the great interpreters of Cole Porter music remaining in this world. "If you're at all intelligent, by the time you're twenty-one you know how much your body can take. I learned about my body a long time ago. The same set of nerves that allow me to perform are also capable of manufacturing an acid which is indigestible, so I must keep those nerves under control."

One way, I should think, would be to live as he lives, in a nine-room apartment in a rambling Victorian building in midtown Manhattan, with a gleamingly lacquered piano here, a wall of mirrors over there, and such assorted objets d'art as a New Guinea ritual-house pole, a West African goat-head carving, and a no-nonsense fireplace in the library, complete with wooden bucket and broom.

Bicycling is the aerobic sport that also helps him unwind. "My doctor says it's either that or tennis or swimming." He has two bikes, French and Japanese. He'll ride two miles downtown for lunch in Greenwich Village or bring his bike on the ferry and ride the hills over on Staten Island.

Short generally eats one big meal a day. "I usually skip dessert, but then once in a while I get crazy and take ice cream or a really rich cake. But I never take sugar in tea or coffee." If he gains weight, "I can lose overnight. It's a matter of discipline. I just eat very little until I lose what I want to lose. I could get along without red meat for the rest of my life."

He stands five feet nine inches but looks taller. He has perfect posture. "I'm addressing the audience when I perform. I have to be in command, don't I? I can't do that and slump. It's a matter of discipline, I guess, and vanity. There are some things we can control.

"I think of myself a lot in a very positive way. I think one is uncertain how one will look and fare at, say, thirty-two. I'm a better person now than I was at thirty-two.

"I wish the major turning points in my career had occurred ten years earlier. Commercial success is but a drop in the bucket. It only occurred the last ten years, and I've been performing since I was twelve. I could have used it perhaps ten years earlier than when it came."

Short has lost some hair on the crown of his head. "A family trait," he says. "I'm totally unconcerned about it except when it makes itself known professionally: movies; television. A bald spot on top is distracting to an audience, tantamount to having your fly open." When appearing in films or television, he asks for full makeup on the back of his head to fill in the balding area.

"The will to keep on doing sometimes eludes us after a while. Not me, thank God. When I was ten years old, I recited a poem at church about the three most important things in a young man's life: mother; country; God. I thought it was very sweet when I recited it. Today I will myself to succeed for myself, my race, my family."

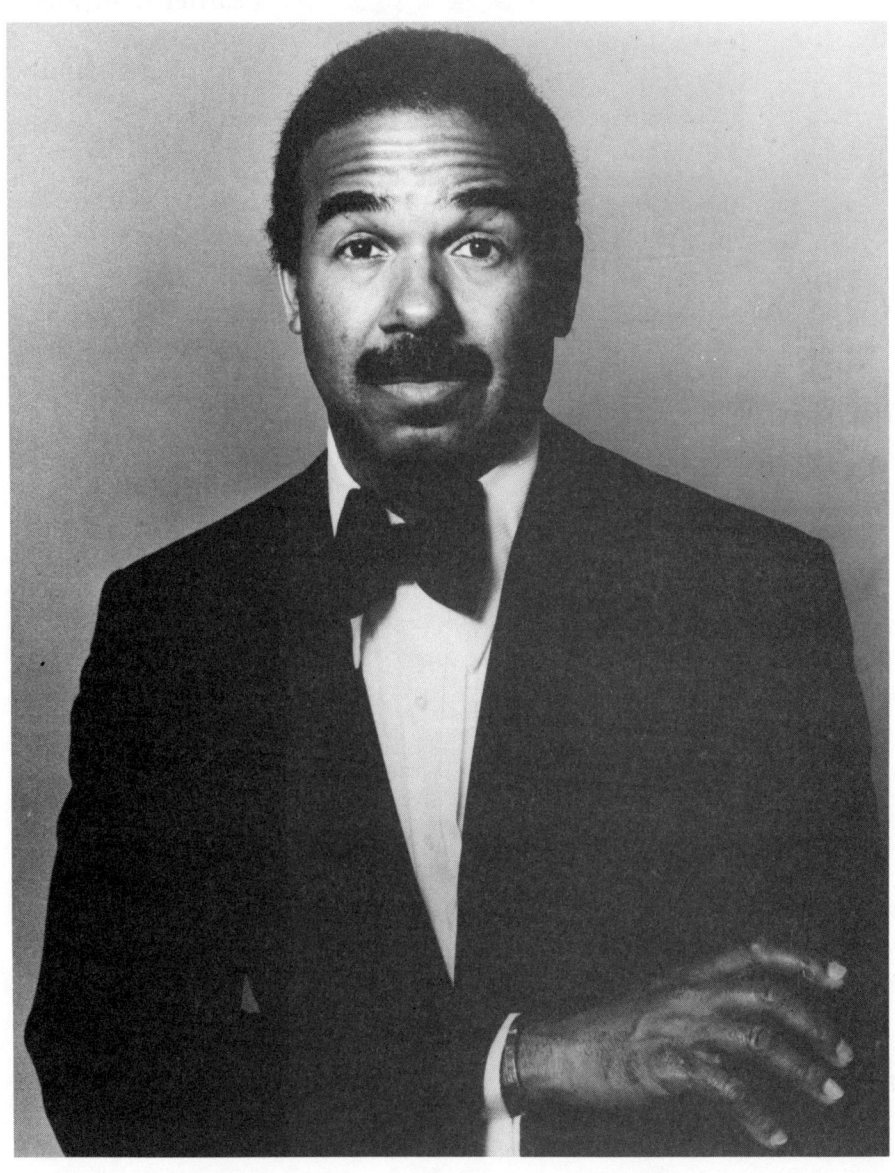

Lowell Thomas

Born 1892

"He communicates a kind of gosh-almighty feeling that the world is his oyster and it contains many nicely turned pearls," *Newsweek* magazine observed back in 1957, when Lowell Thomas was sixty-five. It still applies to this radio pioneer probably heard by more people than any other man in history, whose daily program nowadays is syndicated to several hundred stations coast to coast. He's still a man in perpetual motion, a man who says, "I never go anywhere just for a holiday." His secretary, Electra, who has been with him for nearly half a century, says his schedule never slows down.

I saw him last year at a luncheon meeting of the famous Dutch Treat Club, founded in 1905; he's its eighth president. Hair still thick and wavy, he was nattily turned out in a blue suede jacket and a tie—a gift from Malcolm Forbes—with the words "Capitalist Tool" printed into a neat red design. (Thomas does, after all, own the largest gold mine company in the country.)

His familiar voice still strong and compelling, he spoke wittily, and later I overheard one of the guests regret that he hadn't had a tape recorder with him: "There was magic in the air." Lowell Thomas is still a spellbinder.

He began his career at age eleven, peddling newspapers in the saloons and gambling halls of Colorado's Cripple Creek gold camp, and made his first million writing about a young Oxford archaeologist named T. E. Lawrence, who, as Lawrence of Arabia, was leading the Arabs in battle against their Turkish occupiers. He wrote about him, and "When I found people being so enthralled, I toured the world with a picture-and-word production."

Where does his incredible energy come from? "I've had it all my life," he says. Then, as if to explain further, he adds, "I've always been interested in outdoor activity. I was skiing on my eighty-third birthday; I still play golf; I have an Olympic-sized pool at home but don't get much chance to use it—I'm away so much.

"I've been temperate all my life. I occasionally have one cocktail before dinner. I grew up in a mining town, and I saw so much drink-

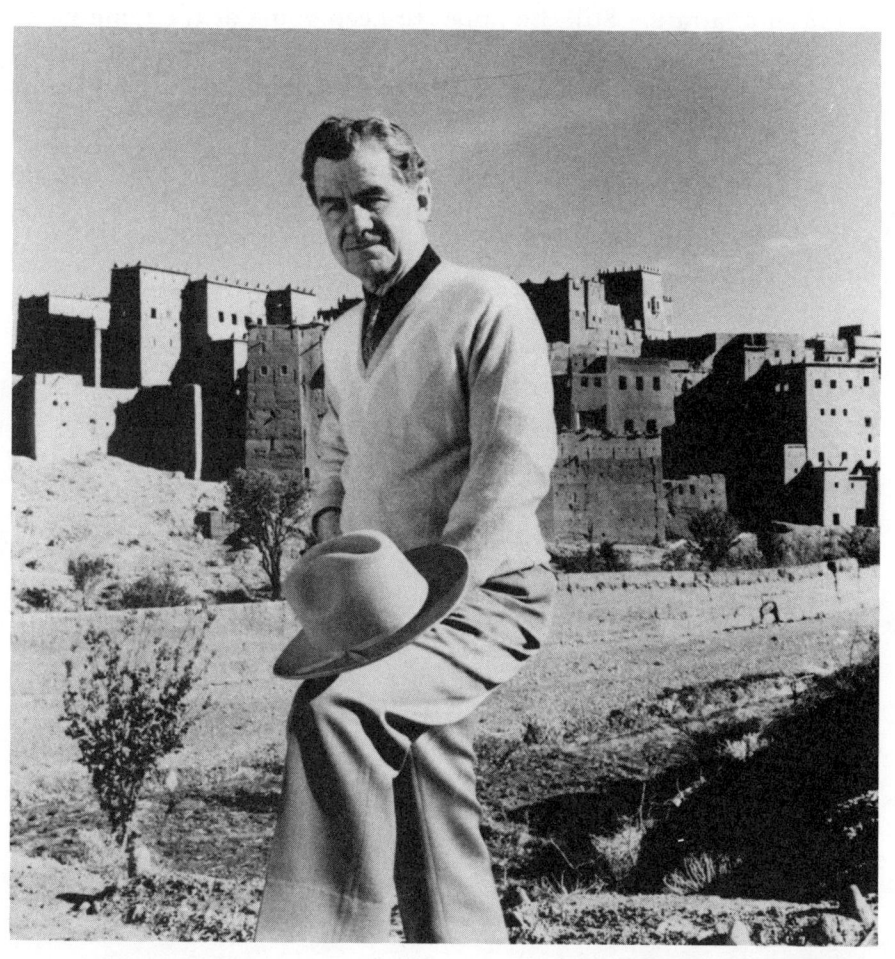

ing as a youngster that it put me off to the point where I'm rather bitter about it." He stopped smoking back in 1914 because it took up too much of his time. But "about once a month," he enjoys a cigar.

He has a mountain range in the Antarctic named after him, and his ambition is still "to know more about this globe than anyone else ever has. But I won't be able to visit any distant planets in my lifetime, I'm afraid." Still, he hopes to keep going at the same pace for another ten years. If he does, he would certainly be the man to send as a sample of one of the more fascinating humans this planet of ours has produced.

John Weitz
Born 1923

"It's difficult for people sometimes to take his self-assurance. He comes on very strong. . . . ." The lady speaking is one of John Weitz's former wives, so she should know. A magazine has referred to his "intimidating 6'2" macho charm," his "glossy image that makes lesser men and women feel gauche." Still another noted: "John Weitz seems to have been born with an uncanny sense of his own destiny." And a female reporter recently decided to dispose of the obvious straightaway in her opening sentence: "First of all, he's terribly good-looking, and not in a fey way."

They're all on target, and Weitz would be the first to say so. A combination of virtuoso design talent and relentless self-promotion has built him a $185 million empire. He designs everything from menswear and women's sportswear to cigars, furniture, eau de cologne, ice buckets, and a spiffy new car called the John Weitz that sells for around $50,000. "It looks as if it were running when it is really standing still," says its creator, sitting at the drawing board in his gray-walled office.

In 1963 Weitz was the first major American designer to enter the menswear field. His label nowadays sells throughout the United States, Canada, Great Britain, and Japan. He so often appears in his own print ads and television commercials that in Japan his face is as well known as that of any movie star. Somehow he also found time a few years ago, while flying between markets, to write a novel that was translated into four languages.

Speaking of his international success and celebrity, Weitz says, "I'm not particularly admiring of the qualities that make me good. You must have the capacity not to need sleep—to consider it a waste of time. You must have a high sense of urgency. All this has to do with some of the worst qualities in a person: impatience; superficiality. You're incapable of wanting to wait and see things happen. It doesn't make for a particularly pleasant person but an avid one."

A former army intelligence officer and amateur race car driver, Weitz nevertheless considers his giving up cigarettes to be "the most macho thing I've ever done. After all, I grew up in an era when it was chic, desirable to smoke; we were taught by the movies that it was sexy. I recall a film with Robert Taylor; he wore a white terrycloth robe and was smoking a cigarette. I thought it looked marvelous. Years later my wife and I had a dinner date with him and his wife; they had to cancel. Bob Taylor was dead of lung cancer one week later."

When Weitz, a three-packs-a-day smoker, stopped smoking, his weight jumped from 190 to 210, and although he hates strenuous exercise, he began doing sit-ups. He got his weight back down. He started with 10, and now he's worked his way up to 180—90 in the morning, 90 in the evening. "Which proves that any idiot thing can be done well."

Weitz has been widely quoted on how a man should look. "Most of all," he says, "a man must always look fit and scrubbed and give the impression that he has just popped out of the shower. And he should wear his clothes as if they are old and valued friends."

He's awesomely efficient. "I'm up at five-thirty, and I'm so furiously organized that I have great blobs of free time." He admits that his design empire is growing almost to a point of absurdity. A camera and refrigerator line may be next. He designs for "the nouveau young—the terribly young, forty- and fifty-year-olds like myself."

How to be a success at whatever you do? Weitz says, "The secret is not to delude yourself that you're doing fine. Instead, propel yourself into instant doom: 'I'm finished. I've lost my touch.'"

How does an overachiever relax? Weitz's lifelong passion is the sea. "It puts things into proportion."

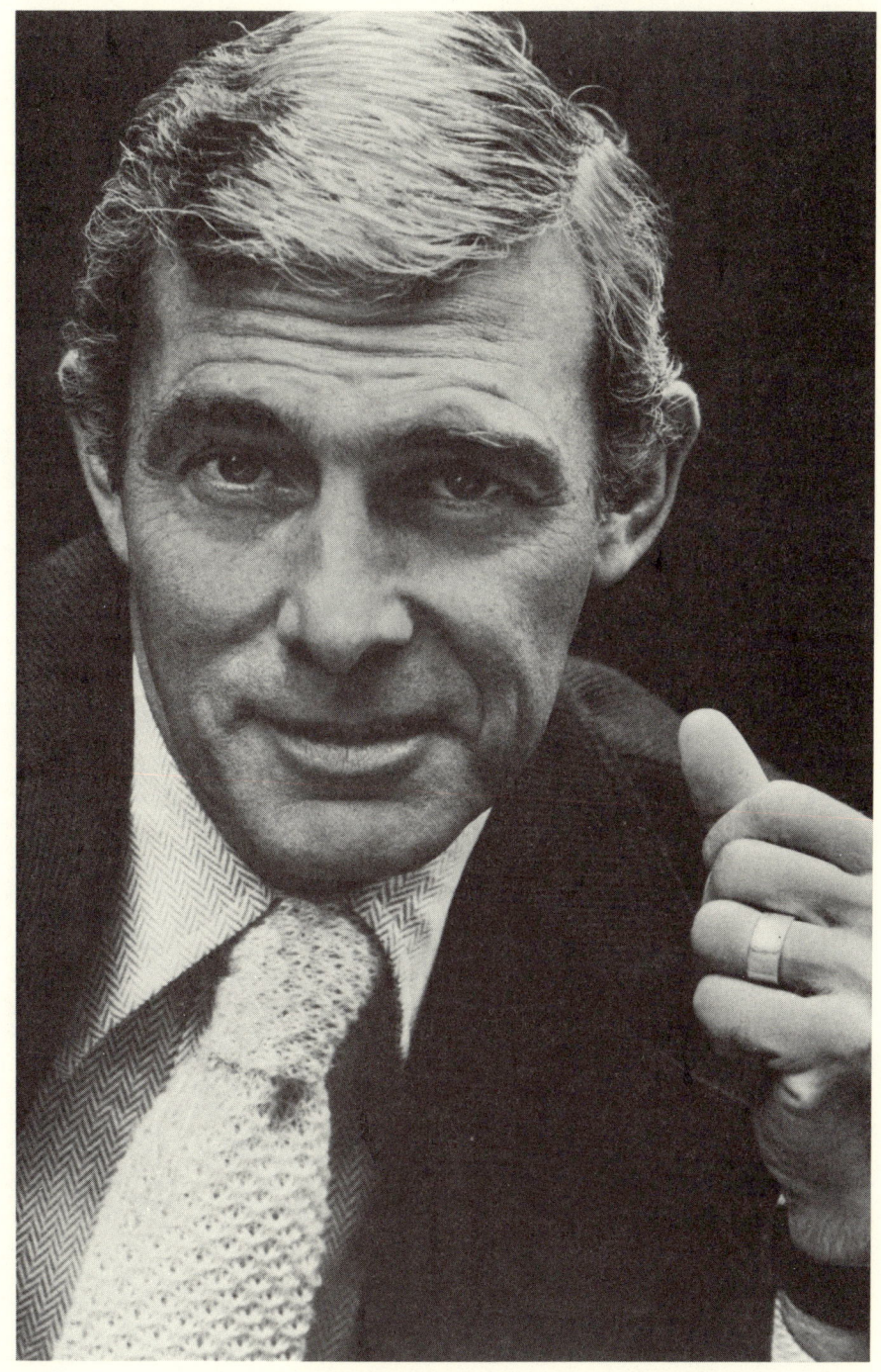

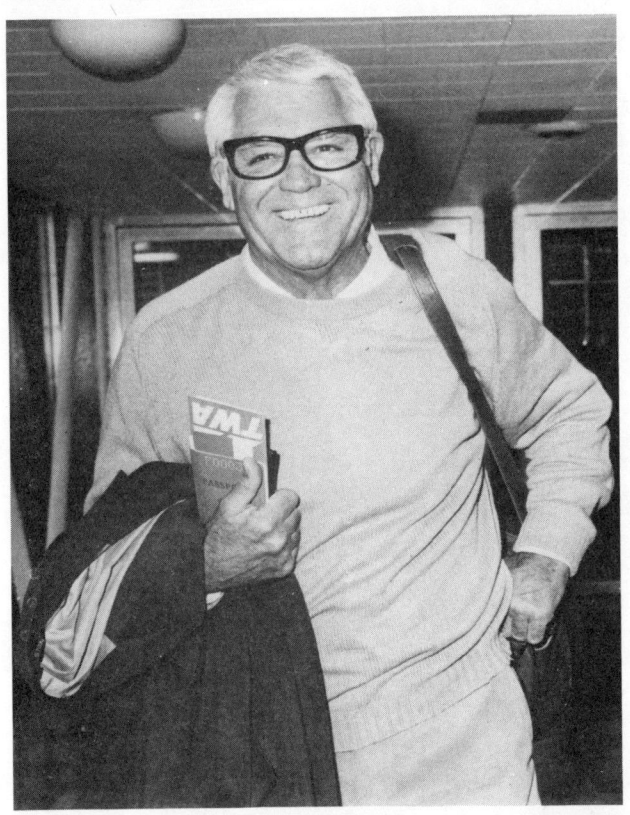

I opened this book with a candid photograph of Cary Grant. So it seems only fitting and proper that I should end it with a comment from the man who holds up his jeans with a belt carrying a buckle proclaiming him to be "Happy Cary."

> My formula for living is quite simple. I get up in the morning, and I go to bed at night. In between, I occupy myself as best I can.

I hope in the pages of this book you've learned some ways to do the same, too, and in the process to look and feel like a million.

—BILL GALE

New York City

Index

Abdomen, exercises for strengthening, 64–65
Acupuncture, cosmetic, 48–50
Acupuncture Treatment Center, 48
Adult males, height and weight standards for, 93
After-shave lotions, 186
Age spots, 74–75
All About Hair (Feinberg), 16
Amies, Hardy, 145, 150, 193–195
Anderson, Warren, 196–197
Aqua Dynamics (exercise program), 121–141
Art of Looking Younger, The (Shelmire), 41
Aslan, Dr. Ana, 51
Asturias, Miguel Angel, 51
Auerbach, Dr. Robert, 47

Back, exercises for strengthening, 64–65
Backaches, prevention of, 61–62
Bad breath, 80
Baker, Jack, 116
Baldness, 25–29
Basketball, 114
Beene, Geoffrey, 162
Berry, Charles, 102
Beverages, recommended servings of, 99–100
Bicycling, 114
Blass, Bill, 149–150, 198–200
Block, Norman, 150
Body hair, excess, 29–30
Bowling, 114
Bread, recommended servings of, 96–97
British warm coats, 177
Bronzers, 39–40
Buf Body Scrub, 34
Bunions, 57
Butler, Jeffrey, 201–203

Calisthenics, 114
Calluses, 57
Canoeing, 115
Cardin, Pierre, 145
Cataracts, 67–68
Cell therapy, 50–52
Cell Therapy Center, 50–51
Cereals, recommended servings of, 96–97
Chain bracelet, 183
Chemabrasion, 46–47

Chesterfield coats, 177
Chin, facial exercises for, 52
Cholesterol, 95
Clinic La Prairie, 50
Clinique's Face Scrub, 34
Coats, 177–179
Colognes, 185–186
Condiments, recommended servings of, 99–100
Conrad, C. Carson, 61, 204–207
Constipation, 103
Contact lenses, 68–70
Corns, 57
Cosmetic acupuncture, 48–50
Cosmetic dentistry, 81
Costill, Dr. David, 111
Cuff links, 183

Dance exercise studios, 117–118
Dancing, 115–116, 118
Dandruff, 21–22
Dardik, Dr. Irving, 108, 111
Davis, Adelle, 94
De Leon, George, 17
Dental floss, 78–79
Dentistry
  cosmetic, 81
  preventive, 76
Dermabrasions, 47
Desserts, recommended servings of, 99–100
DeVries, Dr. Herbert, 110
Diet, well-balanced, 100–103
Dihydrotesterone (DHT), 25–26
Dinner jackets, 168–171
Dress for Success (Molloy), 162
Dried beans, recommended servings of, 95–96
Dry, chapped lips, 81
Dry skin, 31–34
Dunhill Tailors, 150

Eggs, recommended servings of, 95–96
Endo-Stat, 174
Epidermabrasion, 34
Esquire, 159, 168, 181
Evening clothes, 168–171
Exercise studios, 117–118
Exercising, 108–141
  Aqua Dynamics, 121–141
  determining most suitable method of, 113–114

253

INDEX

Exercising (cont.)
  exercise studios, 117–118
  home gymnasium, 117
  rating fourteen sports and exercises, 114
  underrated methods of, 116
  while traveling, 118
Eye-lifts, 71
Eyes, 67–71
  cataracts, 67–68
  contact lenses, 68–70
  dyeing lashes and brows, 71
  glasses, 68–70
  glaucoma, 68
  proper diet for, 67
  red eye, 70–71

Face-lift (rhytidectomy), 44–46
Facial isometrics, 52–53
Facial masks, 35–36
Facials, 37–39
Fad diets, 90
Fairbanks, Douglas, Jr., 208–210
Fairbanks, Paul, 110
Fats, 94–95
  recommended servings of, 98–99
Feet, care of, 56–59
Feinberg, Dr. Herbert S., 16
Fine, William, 211–213
Fingers, exercises for, 75
Fish, recommended servings of, 95–96
Fisher, Dr. Alexander, 33
Fluoride, 79
Food and Drug Administration (FDA), 43, 48, 104, 105
Ford, Eileen, 214
Ford, Gerard William, 214–215
Ford Motor Company, 160
Formal evening wear, 168–169
Fox, Dr. Samuel M., III, 110, 115
Fruit, recommended servings of, 97
Fur coats, 181–183

Gendel, Dr. Evalyn S., 115–116
Gerovital, 51
Gibbs, Dr. Richard, 15, 18, 31–32
Gifford, Frank, 216–218
Giller, Dr. Robert, 16, 85, 106–107
Glasses, 68–70
Glaucoma, 68
Golden Door (health spa), 119
Golf, 114
GQ (Gentlemen's Quarterly), 147
Grant, Cary, 179, 252
Grecian Formula, 16, 24
Greenwood, Dr. Edward, 88
Gwinup, Dr. Grant, 116
Gymnastics, 115–116

H-3, 51–52

Hair, 13–30
  alcohol and, 16–17
  on the body, 29–30
  coloring for, 23–25
  combing and brushing, 19–20
  conditioners for, 20–21
  dandruff, 21–22
  hair weave, 27–28
  haircuts, 22–23
  shampoo, 18–19
Hair dryers, 18–19
Hair implants, 27
Hair transplants, 26–27
Haircuts, 22–23
Hairpieces, 28–29
Handball/squash, 114
Hands, care of, 73–75
Harger, Major Bruce S., 112
Harrison, Rex, 176
Hatfield, Mark, 219–221
Hats, 175–176
Hauser, Gayelord, 56, 94, 222–224
Health spas, 118–119
Health Works '79, 86
Heart rate, maximal, by age, 113
Height and weight standards for adult males, 93
Helmsley, Harry, 120
Henna, 20–21
Herbert, Dr. Victor, 90, 104
Home gymnasiums, 117
Horseback riding, 115
Hosiery, 174–175
Hyman, Stanley, 161

ID bracelets, 183
Isometrics, facial, 52–53

Javits, Jacob, 120
Jawline, the, facial exercises for, 53
Jeans, 179
Jensen, Jim, 225–227
Jewelry, 183
Jogging, 114
Johnson's Odor-Eaters, 59

Kimberly, Jim, 228–230
Knox gelatin, 74
Kraus, Dr. Hans, 65, 111, 115
Kuntzleman, Dr. Charles, 88
Kurtin, Dr. Stephen, 41

Laguna Hills Leisure World, 110
Lamb, Dr. Lawrence E., 115
Laver, James, 145
Laxatives, 103
Leather coats, 177–179
Lefkovitz, Dr. Albert, 42
Lenox Hill Hospital, 108

INDEX

Lenox Hill Hospital's Hypertension Center, 105
LeWinn, Dr. Laurence R., 43, 44, 45
Life, 9, 185
Lips, dry chapped, 81
Loock, Bill, 231–233
Look Younger, Live Longer (Hauser), 222
Lorillard, Griswold, 168
Lubowe, Dr. Irwin I., 43

Macfadden, Bernarr, 13–14
McGregor, Dr. Rob Roy, 54
McLuhan, Marshall, 240
Mahoney, David Joseph, 234–236
Makeup, 39
Males, adult, height and weight standards for, 93
Mallaby, Alexander, 112
Manicures, 73–74
Marsh, Dr. Cyril, 40–41
Maximal heart rate by age, 113
Mayer, Dr. Jean, 95, 106
Meat, recommended servings of, 95–96
Medical facials, 38–39
Megavitamins, 103–104
Menninger Clinic, 88
Metropolitan Life Insurance Company, 93
Milk products, recommended servings of, 98
Minerals, RDA and sources of, 101–102
Moisturizers, 31–33
Molloy, John, 162–163
Mount Sinai Hospital, 41
Mouth, the, facial exercises for, 53
Mouthwashes, 80

Nagler, Dr. Willibald, 61, 64, 117
Nail strengtheners, 74
Nails, 73–75
Navia, Warren M., 105
Neck, the, facial exercises for, 53
New York Hospital-Cornell Medical Center, 43, 61
New York Times, The, 162, 193, 234
New York University Medical School, 33, 47, 111
Newsweek, 246
Nicholas, Dr. James A., 108
Nickolaus Exercise Centers, 117
Niehans, Paul, 50
Nutritionists, 106–107
Nuts, recommended servings of, 95–96

Oils, recommended servings of, 98–99
Orentreich, Dr. Norman, 26, 34–35, 48, 87
Outerwear, 177–179

Packing for traveling, 187–189
Peas, recommended servings of, 95–96

Percy, Charles, 237–239
Plaque, 76
Plastic surgery, 43–48
Polk, Louis, 240–242
Polo coats, 177
Posture, proper, 61–64
Poultry, recommended servings of, 95–96
President's Council on Physical Fitness and Sports, 61, 86, 110, 120, 204
Preventive dentistry, 76
Pritikin, Nathan, 94
Pritikin Diet, 94, 104
Proper posture, 61–64
Prutting, Dr. John, 85, 88, 102
Psychology Today, 17

Raiford, Dr. Morgan B., 67
Relaxing, 87–90
Rivlin, Dr. Richard, 17, 94–95, 100, 106
Robes, 179
Rodin, Dr. Judith, 90
Rope skipping, 116

Sauna, the, 88–89
Schweiker, Richard, 106
Scrimshaw, Dr. Nevin, 90
Semiformal evening wear, 169–171
Sepson, Dr. Ralph, 48–49
Shampoos, 18–19
Shaving, 34–35
Shelmire, Dr. Bedford, Jr., 41
Sherman, Dr. Ronald E., 15
Shirts, 157–161
 coordinating suits, ties, and, 165–168
Shoes, 171–174
Short, Bobby, 243–245
Silicone injections, 47–48
Skating, 114
Skiing, 114
Skin care, 31–53
 bronzers, 39–40
 cell therapy, 50–52
 cosmetic acupuncture, 48–50
 dry skin, 31–34
 facial isometrics, 52–53
 facial masks, 35–36
 facials, 37–39
 makeup, 39
 oily skin, 34
 plastic surgery, 43–48
 rough spots, 34
 shaving, 34–35
 suntans, 39–43
Slippers, 179
Snacks, recommended servings of, 99–100
Socks, 174–175
Softball, 114
Sore feet, 57
Spots, removing, 183–185

INDEX

Stains, removing, 183–185
Stare, Dr. Frederick, 102–103, 104
Stationary bike, 116
Stephan, Peter, 50–51
Stonecypher, Dr. David, 110
Stress, 85–90
 steps in controlling, 86–87
 symptoms of, 86
Sugar, 104–105
Suits, 149–157
 caring for, 156
 coordinating shirts and ties with, 165–168
 for the fat man, 155
 for the short man, 155
 taking your own measurements, 156–157
 for the tall, thin man, 155
Sunblocks, 41–42
Sunglasses, 69
Sunlamps, 42
Sunscreens, 41
Suntans, 40–43
Swimming, 114, 119–120
Swimwear, 181

Teeth
 cleaning, 78–80
 cosmetic dentistry for, 81
 missing teeth, 81–82
 preventive dentistry for, 76
 proper brushing technique, 79–80
 yellow teeth, 80–81
Tender, Loving Cooking (Hauser), 224
Tennis, 114
Thomas, Lowell, 246–248

Ties, 162–165
 coordinating suits, shirts, and, 165–168
Time, 201
Tooth jacketing, 81
Toothbrushes, 79
Trousers, 154
Tuxedos, 168–171

Valium, 86
Varicose veins, 57–58
Vaseline Camphor Ice, 81
Vegetables, recommended servings of, 97
Velvet dinner suits, 171
Vitamins, RDA and sources of, 100–101
Volleyball, 115

W, 148
Walking, 114, 116
Wall Street Journal, 87
Water skiing, 115
Weight and height standards for adult males, 93
Weight lifting, 117
Weitz, John, 145, 163, 249–251
Well-balanced diet, 100–103
Whelan, Dr. Elizabeth, 104
White, Dr. Paul Dudley, 88, 113
Wigs, 29
Windsor, Duke of, 163, 168
Women's Wear Daily, 145–147
Wool coats, 177

Yellow teeth, 80–81
Youthair, 24